CRITICAL THINKING
Developing Skills in Radiography

CRITICAL THINKING
Developing Skills in Radiography

Kathryn S. Durand, RT(R), AS

Former Program Director
School of Radiologic Technology
Current Director
Inservice Education for Radiology
Lawrence and Memorial Hospital
New London, Connecticut

F.A. Davis Company • Philadelphia

F.A. Davis Company
1915 Arch Street
Philadelphia, PA 19103

Printed in the United States of America

Last digit indicates print number: 10 9 8 7 6 5 4 3 2 1

Publisher: Jean-François Vilain
Senior Editor: Lynn Borders Caldwell
Developmental Editor: Crystal Spraggins
Production Editor: Jessica Howie Martin
Cover Designer: Louis J. Forgione

As new scientific information becomes available through basic and clinical research, recommended treatments and drug therapies undergo changes. The author and publisher have done everything possible to make this book accurate, up to date, and in accord with accepted standards at the time of publication. The author, editors, and publisher are not responsible for errors or omissions or for consequences from any application of the book, and make no warranty, expressed or implied, in regard to the contents of the book. Any practice described in this book should be applied by the reader in accordance with professional standards of care used in regard to the unique circumstances that may apply in each situation. The reader is advised always to check product information (package inserts) for changes and new information regarding dose and contraindications before administering any drug. Caution is especially urged when using new or infrequently ordered drugs.

Library of Congress Cataloging-in-Publication Data

Durand, Kathryn S., 1955–
Critical thinking : developing skills in radiography / Kathryn S. Durand.
p. cm.
Includes bibliographical references and index.
ISBN 0–8036–0343–6
1. Radiography, Medical—Case studies. 2. Problem solving. 3. Competency based education. I. Title.
[DNLM: 1. Radiography. 2. Decision Making. WN 200 D948c 1999]
RC78.15.D87 1999
616.07′572—dc21
DNLM/DLC
for Library of Congress 98–32464
CIP

This book is lovingly dedicated to my parents,
Elaine R. Suplicki and the late Stanley E. Suplicki.

A Note To Educators

As a retired academic program director, I know firsthand how difficult it is to maintain a quality program. Throughout the years, first as a Clinical Coordinator and then as Program Director, I have had to adjust my curriculum to meet the needs of the advancing standards of radiologic technology. During my tenure as program director, all of my students from Lawrence and Memorial Hospital School of Radiologic Technology passed the ARRT examination on the first attempt with grades of which I am proud.

ACCREDITATION STANDARDS

In an effort to maintain a quality program, I began my tenure as program director using the Essentials and then adopted the Standards (when they replaced the Essentials), provided by the Joint Review Committee on Education in Radiologic Technology (JRCERT). Although the original Essentials were sufficient and appropriate in their time, the newer Standards more readily address the changing role of the radiographer in a vastly changed healthcare environment. The JRCERT has provided the leadership and guidance that I believe is necessary to maintain a high quality, state-of-the-art program and has readily adapted to changing times. I have written this book in an effort to share with you some of the techniques that I have used to make my program so successful. I do not claim that these techniques will guarantee success for all students in all programs, but I do know that my former students, now registered radiographers, have a solid base of academic skills, as well as common sense and the ability to make good clinical decisions. I firmly believe that if I or a member of my family were one of their patients, we would be in excellent hands. They are outstanding radiographers.

This material was developed in an effort to provide the students with a solid grounding in critical thinking skills and abilities. The following is a description of how you, the instructor, can integrate this material into your current curriculum. This book should be viewed as an adjunct to your present course structure rather than a separate course unto itself. Present courses such as Anatomy/Physiology, Radiographic Positioning, Radiographic Technique, Medical Ethics, and Patient Care Procedures can benefit from the addition of the material contained herein.

HOW THIS BOOK CAN HELP YOU FULFILL ACCREDITATION STANDARDS

This material can provide a program with quantifiable measurements of students' abilities. These measurements, in turn, can be used by a program to help demonstrate compliance with the following JRCERT Standards for an accredited educational program in radiologic sciences:

Standard One—Mission Goals (Objective 1.5)

What the Standard says:

Assures the program's mission statement and/or goals include measurable student learning outcomes

How this book can help:

By integrating the case studies, performance case studies, and film critique portions of the book into your curriculum and using the suggested measurement techniques provided, your program should be able to document and demonstrate certain measurable student learning outcomes. Although this book can help you provide this type of documentation, it is not intended as a substitute or replacement for a program mission statement/goals. To fulfill this Standard, the methodology that you choose to incorporate into your curriculum should be detailed in your program's mission statement goals.

Standard Three—Organization and Administration (Objective 3.12)

What the Standard says:

Assures periodic evaluation of the curriculum to promote student competence in cognitive, psychomotor and affective domains and problem-solving skills

How this book can help:

This book is specifically designed to provide students with a structured methodology for problem solving. Although the book is written for student radiographers, the problem-solving methods employed herein can be transferred to any situation. This book is designed to help foster a student's growth in problem-solving abilities. Use of the methodology in this book may help a program to provide documentation of compliance with the problem-solving skills portion of this objective. It is important to note that use of the methodology contained herein does not demonstrate that the program is performing periodic evaluations of the curriculum.

Standard Four—Curriculum and Academic Practices (Objectives 4.3, 4.5, 4.8)

What the Standard says:

Objective 4.3-Provides a well structured competency-based curriculum reflecting assessment of the affective, cognitive and psychomotor domains.

Objective 4.5-Documents curriculum content to prepare the student to practice in the professional discipline which includes but is not limited to, oral and written communication, Anatomy and Physiology, Pathology, Patient Care, Radiation Biology and Protection, Medical Ethics and Legal Issues, Application of Radiologic Sciences Theory and Techniques, Quality Assessment, and Competency-Based Clinical Education.

Objective 4.8-Promotes competence in critical thinking and problem-solving skills.

How this book can help:

Standard 4.3 directly calls for a competency-based curriculum. The various sections of this book help to provide student radiographers with realistic simulated situations in which to develop their competency. It also provides the educator with a set of tools to measure that competency. This book can be used as part of your effort to document appropriate curriculum content. Standard 4.8 calls for the promotion (by the program) of both critical thinking and problem-solving skills, which again is what this book is specifically designed to address.

CHAPTER DESCRIPTIONS

Chapter 1: Critical Thinking Skills for Student Radiographers

The first chapter provides your students with the background material needed to make competent, informed clinical decisions. It presents them with a four-step problem-solving approach that is directly related to the clinical decisions that they will need to make. It is designed to prepare students for the clinical experiences presented in Chapter 2.

Chapter 2: Case Studies

This chapter provides students with the opportunity to apply the skills learned in Chapter 1 to various clinical scenarios and situations. This chapter gives your students the opportunity to use their new problem-solving skills in situations that are not life-threatening. Chapter 2 has been designed as a series of work assignments that can be assigned to students and completed off-site. If the educator so chooses, it can easily be incorporated into a formal classroom session. Because this section also contains the author's suggested solutions to the scenarios, students have actually enjoyed the assignments. Following an assignment, I would always try to free up some classroom time to discuss the assignment as a group. The discussions were consistently lively and thoughtful.

Chapter 3: Performance Case Studies for the Laboratory

This chapter takes the information presented in the first two chapters and applies it to a simulated clinical setting. I have attempted to make the settings as realistic as possible in my classes, and have found that doing so provides the students with the necessary skills as well as a well-deserved boost to their confidence. This section should be presented to students who have already met the basic clinical competencies. I prefer to think of this section as an opportunity for students to pull all the information they have learned up to this point together into a more coherent knowledge base. This section gives you a firsthand opportunity to see creative clinical thinking in action. Your clinical instructors can give this presentation to a small group at a time. The forms in this chapter give you the chance to review each student's performance and provide you with documentation that your students have met the outcome assessment requirements of your program. It also provides you with the ability to quickly review each student's workbook and to be immediately informed of each student's abilities.

Chapter 4: Critical Analysis of Radiographs

This chapter is directed at the student who has been determined to be clinically competent and is currently working on critiquing radiographs. So often, students work with a staff radiographer in an environment that makes it difficult to evaluate their work. In this section, students take one of the radiographs that they have completed and critique their work using a clear concise format.

Once again, this does not take time away from your classroom curriculum but rather enhances the information that you and your instructors have already presented. This section gives students the opportunity to review their workbooks periodically to ensure that they are progressing in an acceptable manner. This section gives you the ability to review all of your students' progress without placing an additional burden on your already overwhelming workload.

An Instructor's Guide has been completed to accompany this book. The guide is available in hardcopy and from the F. A. Davis web site (see below).

If you would like additional ideas for critical thinking exercises you can do in the classroom, please visit the "Faculty Lounge" at the F. A. Davis web site, http:\\www.fadavis.com.

Acknowledgments

I could easily double the length of this book by devoting a paragraph each to everyone who has helped me bring it to fruition. However, instead let me say a collective "thank you" to the following people.

- The book reviewers listed on the following pages. Their expertise has been greatly appreciated.

- The staff of F. A. Davis: Crystal Spraggins; Jessica Howie Martin; Samuel Rondinelli; and especially Lynn Borders Caldwell, my editor, for their professionalism and support.

- The radiographers of Lawrence and Memorial Hospital, especially Carol Allen, RT(R); Kris Babbin RT(R); Amy Bjork, RT(R); Bruce Cadieux, RT(R); Barbara Cawley, RT(R)(M); Bill Doak, RT(R); Betty Drew, RT(R)(M); Miranda Eukel, RT(R); Phyllis Jansen, RT(R)(M); Daphne Karnes, RT(R)(M); Melissa Kearney, RT(R); Lewis Lorinsky, RT(R); Donna Morrisette, RT(R); Alison Ozga, RT(R); Kris Powers, RT(R)(M)(CV); Julie Rebein, RT(R); Amy Rezendes, RT(R); Pauline Rocha, RT(R); and Rose Siragusa, RT(R). The entire department was extremely helpful to me, but these radiographers were especially helpful with their knowledge and support.

- The radiologists of Ocean Radiology, particularly Leonard Copertino, MD; John Sutphen, MD; David Hayes, MD; Farouk Soydan, MD; Peter Molloy, MD; Thomas Manning, MD; and Brenda Koblick, MD. Either directly or indirectly, they have had a profound influence on me as a radiographer.

- As you realize if you are a radiography educator or involved with radiography students in any way, these educators are a unique group of individuals. Although I have met and enjoyed exchanging ideas with many of them over the years, I would like to thank Mark Patrous, RT(R); Fran Lutz, RT(R); and Marian Sciacchitano, RT(R) for all their help and inspiration.

- My family has been extremely supportive of this endeavor. My mother-in-law, Elizabeth Durand, has watched Hayley for me while I worked. My son, Zachary, has helped with many computer problems. I truly stand in awe of him. My daughter, Emily, has kept an eye on my desk and kept everyone away from the papers. She has also left me wonderful love notes, which I have found in the most unusual places. I thank my best friend, Tricia Dustin, RT(R)(M), who is like a sister to me, for her unending support and encouragement. I thank my father, the late Stanley Suplicki, for expecting so much, and my mother, Elaine Suplicki for never doubting my abilities. A special thank you to my husband, Don, for standing by me each step of the way. He is my mentor, my best friend, and a true gift.

Reviewers

Mary Jo Bergman, MEd, MS, RN, RT(R)
Program Director–Radiology
Chemical Addiction RN
MedCenter One Health System
Bismarck, North Dakota

William J. Callaway, BA, RT(R)
Director, Radiographic Program
Chair, Allied Health Department
Lincoln Land Community College
Springfield, Illinois

Richard R. Carlton, MS, RT(R), (CV), FAERS
Assistant Professor
Arkansas State University
Radiologic Science and Education
State University, Arkansas

Michele S. Diesen, MS, MA, RT(R)
Instructor/Clinical Coordinator
Radiologic Technology Division
Ohio State University
Columbus, Ohio

Frances Gilman, MS, RT(R), (CT)
Clinical Coordinator
Thomas Jefferson University and
Clinical Instructor
Community College of Philadelphia
Philadelphia, Pennsylvania

Diane M. Kawamura, PhD, RT(R), RDMS
Professor
Radiologic Sciences
Weber State University
Ogden, Utah

Elizabeth W. Price, BS, RT(R), (C), (M)
Director of Radiologic Sciences
Burlington County College
Pemberton, New Jersey

Gary P. Randle, MS, RT(R)
Professor/Program Director
Department of Radiography
Manatee Community College
Bradenton, Florida

Dorothy A. Saia, MA, RT(R)
Director
Radiography Program
The Stamford Hospital
Stamford, Connecticut

Albert M. Snopek, BS, RT(R), (M), (CV)
Assistant Professor
Middlesex County College
Edison, New Jersey

Contents

1

Critical Thinking Skills for Student Radiographers

DEVELOPING CRITICAL THINKING SKILLS

The ability to make clinically accurate decisions is a fundamental requirement for becoming a successful radiographer. Clinical decision making has been defined as "a complex process [with] multiple cue states . . . the processing of a vast amount of information, and uncertainty of the outcomes."[1] The ability to make valid decisions in a clinical setting relies heavily on the individual radiographer's critical thinking skills. Critical thinking has been defined as "the cognitive skills of comprehension, application, analysis, synthesis and evaluation."[2]

It is useful to present the above definition in a more concrete fashion. Therefore, follow the critical thinking steps listed below:

1. Define the goal (evaluation of desired outcome).
2. Note your observations.
3. List possible options and their consequences (related to your observations).
4. Select the best available option.

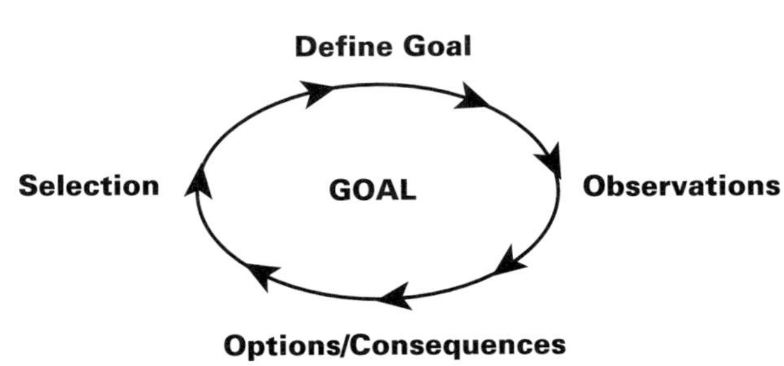

With the above model, the process is implemented in four steps. Each step can be discussed and practiced in class, before using all four in a comprehensive decision-making situation. This model offers radiographers a logical approach to what often appears to be a chaotic clinical situation.

Goals

Simple Goals

A goal is defined as the "end toward which effort is directed."[3] It should be clear from this definition that for an effort to be perceived as useful, it must be directed toward a specific end point. A goal can be simple, short-term, and straightforward, such as "I'm hungry. I will drive to that fast-food restaurant." Being hungry is the problem or situation that needs to be solved, and pulling into the restaurant's parking lot becomes a step toward fulfilling the goal. Individuals tend to approach these types of goals almost "on autopilot." Little conscious thought is given to the steps involved in reaching this goal. Everyone achieves these types of simple goals every day. However, despite the fact that many goals appear simple, there is still a series of steps or plans that collectively contribute to the achievement of the goal. Planning and subsequent goal setting can thus be viewed as a series of actions leading to some type of conclusion.

Complex Goals

A more complex goal involves a series of subgoals. Conscious thought must be applied to the process of completing the subgoals while keeping the final goal in perspective. As a radiography student, you are seeking to acquire the necessary skills to successfully perform diagnostically acceptable radiographs on patients. These skills essentially make up a series of subgoals necessary for you to become a radiographer. However, despite their subordinate nature, each set of subgoals is critical to your ultimate success. Because of the inherent complexity of the ultimate goal (becoming a radiographer), you are forced into a delicate balancing act involving the final goal and the subordinate goals along the way. The final goal should act as a backdrop and a beacon for the set of skills that you must master.

In a complex goal situation, each individual step toward the final result must be assessed, fitted into its proper place in the sequence, and then acted upon. Although there may be a wide range of variability in terms of where a particular subgoal gets placed in the overall sequencing, the subgoals, by default, must be completed successfully before the final goal can be achieved. A complex goal can thus be thought of as a series of smaller goals concluding in a single outcome. Another way of viewing a goal, large or small, is as a problem to be solved. The solution to one problem yields information that may lead to the solution for another problem and so on.

In radiography, the goal is commonly thought to be the radiographic examination itself. An example of a subgoal might be the ability to activate the radiographic equipment. This must be accomplished before completing a radiographic examination. If it is not possible to energize the equipment, the examination cannot be completed. The radiographer now has a new goal, which is to find working equipment that can be used to complete the examination.

It is also a good idea to find out as much as possible as to why an examination has been requested by a physician. The goal of the physician may not be obtainable because of certain circumstances. As a radiographer, you are obligated to help protect the welfare of your patient by suggesting alternatives when necessary. For example, a physician might order a routine os calcis for a stress fracture. In the best interests of your patient, you might suggest to the physician an erect oblique image of the os calcis to best demonstrate the area in question.[4]

Observation

Observation is the "act of noting . . . facts or occurrences."[5] It can be argued that observation should take place before the setting of goals (or solving of problems), but it is difficult or impossible to accurately observe something without having a proper frame of reference (i.e., a goal). The physical act of observing requires that the observer be attentive to the detail surrounding the situation being observed. As humans, we usually seek to fit our current observations into a previously experienced frame of reference. Because a goal is, in essence, a series of problems that need to be solved, we often use our learned experiences (a learned, memorized, working plan or procedure is known as an *algorithm*[6]) when confronted with new goals. In general, we prefer to approach our observations of a goal with learned experiences in mind; however, this is not always possible, and we may have to apply a trial-and-error approach to the problem at hand. A trial-and-error approach is known as *heuristic reasoning*. Although it is more time consuming than the application of a learned experience, a trial-and-error approach may lead to new ways of achieving goals and solving problems. Referring back to the fast-food example, if you always go to a particular restaurant for lunch and order the "Big Burger with Special Sauce," you do so for a number of reasons. You like the taste of the "Big Burger," the service is fast, and the food is of the same consistent quality each time you go. Your repeated trips to this particular restaurant thus become learned experiences (or algorithms). If you find yourself far from home and hungry, you might first attempt to find one of the restaurants that serve the "Big Burger with Special Sauce." If you fail to find one, however, you are then forced into a trial-and-error approach (heuristic reasoning) to satisfy your hunger. If you get lucky and find a place that you like on your first attempt, you will then add that particular experience to your collection of learned experiences, thus reducing your uncertainty in similar future situations.

Ultimately, as humans "we perceive situations as problems, and therefore undertake to solve them."[7] Incorrect observation of a situation can thus lead to the application of incorrect problem-solving skills, which in turn leads to failure to achieve the defined goal. A good example of this would be if you misinterpreted your patient's abilities and had your patient attempt to stand when he was not physically able to do so. Because of your error, your goal has suddenly changed. You are no longer concerned with performing the patient's radiographic examination. Instead, your new goal could be to get medical attention for your patient. For a radiographer, areas of observation should include the following:

- Physical and mental status of the patient
- Needs of the patient (physical and mental)
- Equipment available
- Technical abilities of the equipment

Options and Consequences

When you are preparing to work toward a goal to solve a given problem, various options may present themselves. For example, if you were asked to find the square root of 1849, you could use several methods. You may remember how to perform the long-division method learned in high school to arrive at the answer (algorithm method). If you fail to remember that method, you may use a series of trial-and-error efforts, eventually arriving at the correct response (heuristic reasoning). Or, you may simply enter the number 1849 into your calculator and press the square root key. The choice of method that you use in this example depends on other factors. You may not have a calculator available, and that option is thus closed to you. You may not remember the long-division method *and* not have a calculator available. In that case, your only option is trial and error.

A clinical example of this could involve the use of the inverse square law. A patient needs a chest radiograph, but for reasons beyond your control, the maximum distance that can be obtained in the only room available to you is 40 in. Thus, a change in technique becomes necessary. You could use the inverse-square-law formula (a learned experience) and calculate the exact factors to be used. You could apply a trial-and-error approach and simply decrease the technique by 1 milliampere second (mAs) station or decrease the screen speed while maintaining your original technique settings.

The options that you choose or that are chosen by external factors will lead to differing sets of consequences. Continuing with the first example above, you may be forced to use a trial-and-error method, which can lead to frustration. The frustration, in turn, may cause you to feel that the goal (the square root of 1849) was simply not worth the effort. On the other hand, if you had a calculator, the problem would take no more than a few seconds to solve, and you would then be ready for the next challenge, with minimal frustration. In the clinical example, failure to use the correct technique (derived from the correct use of the inverse square law) would result in increased and unnecessary exposure to the patient and possibly a large number of wasted films. Thus, if there is any semblance of control over the various options, the consequences or outcomes of each option should be carefully weighed before choosing. When listing options, it is best to list all of them, even if you do not find one that is appropriate. This is called *brainstorming.* After each option, write down the consequence(s) of that option. This should help to focus the available options and allow you to zero in on a preferable one.

For example, if your goal is to produce a radiographic examination of the chest taken with the patient erect and the patient is not able to stand, your list of options might appear as follows:

Stand the patient anyway.	Not an option
Complete the examination with the patient sitting.	Possibility
Cancel the examination.	Not an option
Instead of radiographing the patient in the erect position, radiograph the patient in the recumbent position.	Possibility

Selection

The final stage in this process is the selection of a set of options designed to solve the problem or achieve the goal at hand. Consequences must be measured along with each step and choices made based on the anticipated consequences associated with each action. When you are operating in a patient care environment, your assessment of consequences is of the utmost importance. Any single action on your part may have undue consequences for the patient. As a radiographer, you are required to balance the goals of producing a diagnostically acceptable image with those of providing support and physical comfort for the patient in your care. These broad-based goals may be in conflict, and it becomes your task (goal) to balance them and reconcile them so that the patient's physical and diagnostic needs are both met.

Once you have listed your options and reviewed which option or options you feel has or have some chance of success, you must then select the most appropriate one and begin to implement your decision.

References

1. Hammond, BB, et al: Clinical inference in nursing. Nurs Res 15:134, 1996.
2. Matthews, CA, and Gaul, AL: Nursing diagnosis from the perspective of concept attainment and critical thinking. Advances in Nursing Science, 1979, 17.

3. Morris, W (ed): The American Heritage Dictionary of the English Language. Houghton Mifflin, Boston, 1980, 564.
4. Ballinger, PW: Merrill's Atlas of Radiographic Positions and Radiologic Procedures, ed 8, Vol 1. Mosby, St. Louis, 1995, p 219.
5. Morris, op cit, p 906.
6. Hunt, M: The Universe Within. Simon and Schuster, New York, 1982, p 83.
7. Ibid, p 129.

Bibliography

Ballinger, PW: Merrill's Atlas of Radiographic Positions and Radiologic Procedures, ed 8, Vols 1–3. Mosby, St. Louis, 1995.

Hammond, BB, et al: Clinical Inference in Nursing, Nurs Res, 15:134, 1966.

Hunt, M: The Universe Within. Simon and Schuster, New York, 1982.

Matthews, CA, and Gaul, AL: Nursing Diagnosis from the Perspective of Concept Attainment and Critical Thinking. Advances in Nursing Science, 1979, p 17.

Morris, W (ed): The American Heritage Dictionary of the English Language. Houghton Mifflin, Boston, 1980.

2

Case Studies

Cases

- Case 2.1: Skull Positioning
- Case 2.2: Hand (Extremity) Positioning
- Case 2.3: Positioning in Trauma
- Case 2.4: Bony Thorax Positioning
- Case 2.5: Positioning for the Gastrointestinal Examination
- Case 2.6: Locating a Foreign Body
- Case 2.7: Positioning in Surgery
- Case 2.8: Confidentiality in Patient Care
- Case 2.9: The Geriatric Patient
- Case 2.10: The Pediatric Patient
- Case 2.11: The Psychotic Patient
- Case 2.12: The Patient in Trauma
- Case 2.13: The Paraplegic Patient
- Case 2.14: The Patient Who Refuses an Examination
- Case 2.15: The Patient with Alzheimer's Disease
- Case 2.16: Soft Tissue
- Case 2.17: Trauma Exposure Techniques
- Case 2.18: High-kVp Techniques in GI Examinations
- Case 2.19: Manual versus Automatic Exposure Techniques
- Case 2.20: Multiproblematic: The Pediatric Patient in Trauma
- Case 2.21: Multiproblematic: Barium Enema Examination for a Geriatric Patient
- Case 2.22: Multiproblematic: The Pregnant Patient in Trauma
- Case 2.23: Multiproblematic: Lack of Radiation Protection in a Trauma Situation
- Case 2.24: Multiproblematic: The Pediatric Patient with Multiple Trauma
- Case 2.25: Multiproblematic: Radiation Protection in Surgery and the Unreasonable Orthopedist

Author's Opinions

CASES

In this chapter, read each case study, then write your goal, your observations, and what you think are the options and their consequences in the spaces provided. Use and attach extra paper if needed. Compare your answers to those suggested in Selection of the Best Option and in the Author's Opinions following the case studies. Be prepared to discuss your answers in class.

Case 2.1 Skull Positioning

➤ Prerequisites

Before attempting this case study, the student should be knowledgeable of[1]:

- Positioning for skull examinations
- Trauma radiography
- Skull anatomy

DESCRIPTION ➤➤ Your patient is a 35-year-old man with very large shoulders. He has sustained a direct trauma to the frontal area of his skull caused by bricks falling off a scaffold and striking him on the head. The physician in charge has ordered a skull series, consisting of a posteroanterior (PA) skull and bilaterals. Because of the patient's injuries, he cannot lie in the prone position and has great difficulty keeping the back of his head on the radiographic table while trying to depress his chin. To assist your patient, you place a radiolucent sponge under his head. Even with the sponge in place, the patient's orbitomeatal line is not perpendicular to the cassette top. You decide to complete the examination, hoping that the image is acceptable. On inspection of the reverse PA skull radiograph, you notice that the orbits are very round and only a small portion of petrous ridge can be seen in the lower edge of the orbit. The lateral images appear to be acceptable. What do you do about the reverse PA skull radiograph?

➤ Identify the Following

GOAL

OBSERVATIONS

OPTIONS AND CONSEQUENCES

➤ Selection of the Best Option

GOAL

To submit a skull examination that is diagnostically acceptable.

OBSERVATIONS

The reverse PA skull image does not demonstrate structures that should be seen on this image.

OPTIONS AND CONSEQUENCES

Option 1

You decide to submit the poorly positioned reverse PA skull image. You think that this is the best image that you can obtain because of the patient's condition.

Consequence

Given the patient's condition, this may be true.

Option 2

You decide to take another reverse PA skull radiograph. Because you were able to demonstrate a small portion of the petrous ridges on the lower border of the orbit, you may be able to demonstrate more by angling the central ray caudally.

Consequence

Increased radiation exposure to the patient.

Case 2.2 Hand (Extremity) Positioning

➤ Prerequisites

Before attempting this case study, the student should be knowledgeable of[2–6]:

- Hand positioning
- Skeletal anatomy
- The placement of the central ray
- Adaptation of positions because of patient's condition
- Pathology in relation to positioning

DESCRIPTION ➤➤ Your patient is a 35-year-old man who has rheumatoid arthritis of both hands. He recently injured both hands during a fall. You have been asked to radiograph each hand and each wrist. As you prepare to radiograph the patient's hands, you notice that he is unable to straighten his fingers. You also notice that the skin on both hands appears very taut. It is obvious that straightening them will not be an option. What do you decide is the best way to position his hands?

➤ Identify the Following

GOAL

OBSERVATIONS

OPTIONS AND CONSEQUENCES

➤ Selection of the Best Option

GOAL

To obtain the best diagnostic radiographs possible under the circumstances.

OBSERVATIONS

The patient is unable to straighten his fingers and place his hand flat.

OPTIONS AND CONSEQUENCES

Option 1

For the PA projection, place the patient's hand as flat as possible on the cassette. Radiograph each hand separately. Proceed with the routine oblique and lateral radiographs. Use radiographic sponges as necessary to help hold the positions.

Consequence

Distortion may be seen in the phalanges on the PA projection.

Option 2

For the PA projections, radiograph the hands as flat as possible on the cassette. For the oblique positions, place both of the patient's hands in a semiprone position. The phalanges will be slightly curled in this position because of the tightness of the skin on the patient's hand. Proceed with the routine lateral radiographs.

Consequence

The semiprone oblique position of the hands will not demonstrate the interphalangeal joints as well.

Option 3

For the PA projections, radiograph the hand in the supine position (anteroposterior [AP] hands and fingers). Take two exposures of each hand. For the metacarpal area, direct the central ray to the palm of the patient's hand. To demonstrate the phalangeal area, place the supinated hand on the cassette and roll the hand until the phalanges are nearly parallel with the cassette. Direct the central ray perpendicular to the film, approximately at the level of the interphalangeal joint of the third phalanx. This, along with the AP metacarpal position, should demonstrate the entire hand. For the oblique positions, you might want to position the hand in the AP oblique position as described in the AP oblique position (Norgaard method).[2] Proceed with routine lateral radiographs.

Consequence

The AP 45-degree oblique position (Norgaard method) will demonstrate the metacarpal heads and early stages of rheumatoid arthritis.

Case 2.3 Positioning in Trauma

➤ Prerequisites

Before attempting this case study, the student should be knowledgeable of[7]:

- Positioning all possible radiographic examinations satisfactorily
- Adjusting standard positions to accommodate the involved trauma
- Skeletal anatomy
- How to plan and organize a trauma examination in an efficient manner (i.e., radiographing the most important area first)

DESCRIPTION ➤➤ Your patient is a 22-year-old man who comes to the trauma center with injuries from a motorcycle accident. The following examinations have been requested:

Femurs (bilateral)
Pelvis
Lumbar spine
Right lower leg
Right foot

On receiving the requisition, you begin to organize and obtain the equipment needed. This includes gloves, goggles, protective face shield, eyewear, lead aprons, and cassettes. The nurse informs you that the patient's main injuries seem to be in the pelvic region and that the patient is having dyspnea. You quickly write down the examinations requested in the order in which you feel they can be most efficiently performed. You also suspect that the physician in charge will probably want abdomen and chest radiographs as well. What do you do?

➤ Identify the Following

GOAL

OBSERVATIONS

OPTIONS AND CONSEQUENCES

➤ Selection of the Best Option

GOAL

To perform the examinations in the most efficient manner possible, starting with the most diagnostically important area.

OBSERVATIONS

The patient is in considerable pain, with possible life-threatening injuries. The physician has not yet ordered a chest and abdomen series.

OPTIONS AND CONSEQUENCES

Option 1

First, ask the doctor if radiographs of the chest and abdomen are going to be ordered. You decide to start at the top of the patient (literally) and work your way down, completing each examination in order. The following is the order in which the examinations will be performed:

Chest
Abdomen (this includes the AP lumbar spine)
Pelvis
Lateral lumbar spine
AP right femur
Lateral right femur
AP left femur
Lateral left femur
AP right tibia
Lateral right tibia
AP right foot
Lateral right foot

Consequence

This sequence of examinations will complete the required list of radiographs.

Option 2

The physician has confirmed that radiographs of the chest and abdomen are also requested. The following is the order in which the examinations will be performed:

AP chest
AP abdomen (including lumbar spine)
AP pelvis
AP right and left femurs
AP right tibia
AP right foot
Lateral lumbar spine (right lateral)
Lateral right femur
Lateral right tibia
Lateral right foot
Lateral left tibia

Consequence

This sequence of examinations will complete the required list of radiographs.

Case 2.4 Bony Thorax Positioning

➤ Prerequisites

Before attempting this case study, the student should be knowledgeable of[8–11]:

- Positioning the bony thorax satisfactorily
- Bony thorax anatomy
- Adjusting routine positioning if necessary
- Exposure techniques relating to pathological changes

DESCRIPTION ➤➤ Your patient is an obese 68-year-old woman who has been in an automobile accident. She has sustained injuries to her chest caused by the steering wheel. She has been transported to the x-ray room via stretcher and is unable to stand. The patient states that she is able to sit, and the patient's nurse has approved this. The physician has ordered radiographs of the bilateral ribs and sternum. You decide that you will take all of the radiographs with the patient seated, using an upright grid.

On review of the radiographic images, you find that all of the images are acceptable, with the exception of the lateral sternum. The sternum is not demonstrated well because of the woman's large breasts and upper arm flesh. What do you do?

➤ Identify the Following

GOAL

OBSERVATIONS

OPTIONS AND CONSEQUENCES

➤ Selection of the Best Option

GOAL

To demonstrate the sternum free of soft tissue obstruction to the extent allowed by the patient's condition.

OBSERVATIONS

Because of soft tissue obstruction of the patient's breasts, as well as her fleshy upper arms, her sternum is not well demonstrated.

OPTIONS AND CONSEQUENCES

Option 1

Position the patient in the recumbent supine position (dorsal decubitus position). Allow the breasts to fall laterally. Radiograph the patient using a horizontal central ray.

Consequence

This position should allow less soft tissue obstruction and better visualization of the sternum.

Option 2

You repeat the erect lateral radiograph with an increase in peak kilovolts (kVp).

Consequence

Increasing kVp will increase the penetrability of the beam, possibly allowing penetration of the patient's fleshy masses and demonstrating the lateral sternum.

Case 2.5 Positioning for the Gastrointestinal Examination

➤ Prerequisites

Before attempting this case study, the student should be knowledgeable of[12]:

- Positioning patients satisfactorily for upper gastrointestinal (UGI) examinations
- Anatomy of the GI system
- The use of contrast media

DESCRIPTION ➤➤ Your patient has arrived for his UGI series and the procedure begins. The patient thoroughly dislikes the taste of the barium. In fact, you have had to coax him to drink the little he has had so far. You know how important barium is for this study. Halfway through the fluoroscopic examination, the radiologist tells you that the patient has hypermotility of the GI tract. You are to give the patient more barium before each exposure is taken. The radiologist completes her portion of the examination, leaving the patient in the right anterior oblique (RAO) position on the radiographic table. As you begin to prepare for your overhead radiographs, the patient continues to complain about drinking the barium. What do you do?

➤ Identify the Following

GOAL

OBSERVATIONS

OPTIONS AND CONSEQUENCES

➤ Selection of the Best Option

GOAL

To obtain a successful study by having the patient drink as little barium as possible.

OBSERVATIONS

The patient has already complained about the amount of barium he has had to drink. The stomach empties very fast. The radiologist has left the patient in an RAO position.

OPTIONS AND CONSEQUENCES

Option 1

Take the time to explain once again how important it is for the patient to drink barium. Explain to the patient that he has the right to refuse the examination.

Consequence

The patient may refuse the examination.

Option 2

Turn the patient to the left posterior oblique (LPO) position and quickly prepare the room. Have everything ready, including the barium. Explain to the patient that you are doing everything that you possibly can to have him drink the least amount of barium that will produce a successful study.

Consequence

If the patient is placed in the LPO position, the barium will fill the fundus and body of the stomach. The duodenum and pylorus are elevated and therefore will not fill with barium. Also, the barium will not empty from the stomach, negating the examination.

Option 3

Give the patient a water-soluble iodinated contrast medium to drink. This does not have the same texture or taste as barium.

Consequence

A water-soluble iodinated contrast medium does not have the same mucosal coating properties as barium.

Case 2.6 Locating a Foreign Body

➤ Prerequisites

Before attempting this case study, the student should be knowledgeable of[13–15]:

- Positioning the forearm
- Positioning for foreign bodies
- Vascular anatomy
- The use of Standard Precautions*

DESCRIPTION ➤➤ Your patient is a 27-year-old man who is a known intravenous (IV) substance abuser. He has presented himself in the emergency department (ED) with the complaint of a possible foreign body in his left forearm. He states that, while he was injecting himself, the needle broke off. He also states that he attempted to retrieve the needle fragment with a knife, but was unsuccessful. His arm has been cut and is bleeding. The physician has ordered a left forearm examination. You successfully complete the examination, using Standard Precautions. The ED is extremely busy. On viewing the radiographs, you see that the needle is not present. To be as efficient as possible, what action do you take?

➤ Identify the Following

GOAL

OBSERVATIONS

OPTIONS AND CONSEQUENCES

*Standard Precausions are found in Draft Guideline for Infection Control in Health Care Personnel (Centers for Disease Control). Federal Register 62(173):47275–47327.

➤ Selection of the Best Option

GOAL

To complete the examination as requested.

OBSERVATIONS

The patient's arm is bleeding. The needle fragment was not demonstrated radiographically on the images of the forearm.

OPTIONS AND CONSEQUENCES

Option 1

You use Standard Precautions when radiographing the patient's forearm. On viewing the images of the left forearm, you observe that the needle fragment is not present. You feel that, to give this patient the best care possible, it would be advisable to x-ray his chest on the chance that the fragment has moved to that area. On viewing the chest radiograph, you see the needle fragment. You immediately inform the patient's physician and give him the radiographs.

Consequence

The needle fragment has been located.

Option 2

You x-ray the patient using Standard Precautions. You immediately give the patient's physician the radiographs of the patient's forearm. You ask him if he would like additional radiographs of the patient's humerus and chest.

Consequence

The patient's physician must determine the next course of action.

Case 2.7 Positioning in Surgery

➤ Prerequisites

Before attempting this case study, the student should be knowledgeable of[16,17]:

- Performing radiographic examinations in the surgical suite
- The use of the C-arm
- Anatomy

DESCRIPTION ➤➤ You are in the surgical suite using the C-arm for insertion of an infusion port catheter. It is your responsibility to fluoroscope the patient's chest while the physician inserts the catheter into the subclavian vein, through the patient's superior vena cava, and finally into the right atrium. The case is proceeding as expected. The C-arm (portable fluoroscopy unit) is in position over the patient's upper abdomen, as requested by the physician. You have not yet fluoroscoped. The C-arm is energized and all room personnel are protected with lead. You are on standby. The physician suddenly asks for fluoroscopy. You begin to fluoroscope, but you are not able to see the catheter. You quickly look at the monitor and try to move the C-arm over the area of interest. You are still unable to locate the catheter tip. At this point, the physician becomes impatient. You continue to move the C-arm more into the chest area, but you are still not over the catheter. You begin to panic. The physician suddenly states, "Get someone in here who knows what he's doing!" What do you do?

➤ Identify the Following

GOAL

OBSERVATIONS

OPTIONS AND CONSEQUENCES

➤ Selection of the Best Option

GOAL

To demonstrate the catheter tip under fluoroscopy.

OBSERVATIONS

The physician has requested that the C-arm be set up over the patient's abdomen. You are not aware of the approximate position of the catheter. The physician is impatient.

OPTIONS AND CONSEQUENCES

Option 1

You immediately have the radiographer take over.

Consequence

You lose your confidence.

Option 2

Immediately after the physician requests fluoroscopy, ask him to approximate where the catheter tip is located. Move the unit to this area.

Consequence

You should locate approximately the area of interest.

Option 3

You tell the physician that you know what you are doing and calmly ask him for the approximate location of the catheter.

Consequence

You should locate approximately the area of interest.

Case 2.8 Confidentiality in Patient Care

➤ Prerequisites

Before attempting this case study, the student should be knowledgeable of[18]:

- Medical ethics
- Positioning abdomen radiographs
- Radiation protection for pregnant women

DESCRIPTION ➤➤ You are working in the ED, and you have just received a requisition for an abdomen series on a patient with severe abdominal pain. The patient is a 26-year-old woman whose name you recognize because she works in the radiology department as a clerk. You have heard rumors that she is having an affair with someone in the hospital and that she is pregnant. The radiographer with whom you are working is currently out of the department, performing a portable examination. According to department policy, you ask the patient the date of her last menstrual period. She says that it was more than a month ago. You ask her if there is any chance that she may be pregnant. She states that she had an abortion and she is no longer pregnant. You proceed with the examination according to department policy, completing the procedure.

You are expecting the radiographer with whom you are working to return within minutes. You will not be discussing this examination with her, but there is a possibility that she could see the radiographs. The radiographs are left on the view box for the physician to view. (This is standard procedure in the emergency department.) What do you do?

➤ Identify the Following

GOAL

OBSERVATIONS

OPTIONS AND CONSEQUENCES

➤ Selection of the Best Option

GOAL

To keep the patient's information confidential.

OBSERVATIONS

The patient's radiographs will be on the view box. The films will be available for the other radiographer to see. The patient identification markers on the films are small and may not be noticed. When you enter the required information into the department computer, the department secretaries will have full access to the data.

OPTIONS AND CONSEQUENCES

Option 1

Do not display your patient's radiographs in your work area. Bring them to the physician and tell him or her that you are doing this to maintain patient confidentiality. Make certain that all patient identification cards are discarded properly and promptly. Give the patient as much privacy as possible. You do not report that the patient stated that she had an abortion when you enter the required information on the computer.

Consequence

You have done everything that you can do to ensure the patient's confidentiality.

Option 2

Follow all hospital and departmental protocols. Be sure not to discuss the information with anyone. The other radiographer is a professional. If she accidentally acquires information, it is up to her not to discuss it. Leave the films in the regular viewing area. (This is the ED's standard protocol.) The identification markers are very small and will probably not be noticed. With regard to the entry in computer, you trust the department secretaries to be professional.

Consequence

You have done everything possible, while following standard protocols, to ensure the patient's confidentiality.

Case 2.9 The Geriatric Patient

➤ **Prerequisites**

Before attempting this case study, the student should be knowledgeable of[19]:

- Satisfactory positioning for chest radiographs
- Geriatric care
- The relationship of the placement of the central ray in regard to radiographic distortion

DESCRIPTION ➤➤ Your patient is an ambulatory 76-year-old woman with extreme kyphosis. Her physician has ordered a chest radiograph. As you begin to position the patient for the PA projection of her chest, you notice that the distance between her chest and the upright grid is considerable. Her kyphosis and her limited ability to lift her chin cause this distance. What will you do to best demonstrate the patient's chest?

➤ **Identify the Following**

GOAL

OBSERVATIONS

OPTIONS AND CONSEQUENCES

➤ Selection of the Best Option

GOAL

To demonstrate the patient's chest area with a minimal amount of distortion.

OBSERVATIONS

The patient is scarcely able to lift her chin and is extremely kyphotic. The object film distance between the patient and the upright grid is considerable.

OPTIONS AND CONSEQUENCES

Option 1

Do not have the patient lift her chin. This will only accentuate the object film distance. Direct the central ray perpendicular. Have the patient stand as relaxed as possible. Explain the circumstances of the case by including a note to the radiologist with the requisition.

Consequence

Although the radiograph is suboptimal, it is the best radiograph that can be obtained under the circumstances.

Option 2

Turn the patient so that her back is against the upright grid. Ask the patient to lift her chin as much as possible. Direct the central ray cephalic.

Consequence

There will be an increase in distortion because of the angled central ray.

Case 2.10 The Pediatric Patient

➤ Prerequisites

Before attempting this case study, the student should be knowledgeable of[20–22]:

- Pediatric radiography
- Pediatric pathologies
- Pediatric anatomy

DESCRIPTION ➤➤ Your patient is a 3-year-old girl who has been brought into the ED by her mother. She has a diagnosis of croup and is having difficulty breathing. This is noted on the patient's requisition. The physician in charge has ordered a chest radiograph. You learn from the patient's mother that the patient is not able to stand. She is currently in a sitting position. What do you do in preparation for her examination?

➤ Identify the Following

GOAL

OBSERVATIONS

OPTIONS AND CONSEQUENCES

➤ Selection of the Best Option

GOAL

Obtain a chest radiograph of a pediatric patient.

OBSERVATIONS

The patient has croup and is not able to stand. She is presently sitting.

OPTIONS AND CONSEQUENCES

Option 1

You decide that you will perform both radiographs of the patient in the sitting position, and you prepare accordingly. These radiographs will demonstrate the presence of fluid in her chest.

Consequence

This procedure should produce diagnostically acceptable radiographs of the chest.

Option 2

You decide that you should use larger cassettes, and prepare accordingly. This option will allow the neck area to be demonstrated on both radiographs. The exposure should be taken at the end of inspiration.

Consequence

This option will demonstrate not only the patient's lungs but the size of the airway as well.

Case 2.11 The Psychotic Patient

➤ Prerequisites

Before attempting this case study, the student should be knowledgeable of[23]:

- Communicating with a psychotic patient
- Positioning

DESCRIPTION ➤➤ You are in the ED. Your patient is a 55-year-old woman with a history of mental illness. The police found her walking in the middle of the road, arguing with an imaginary partner. The police have brought the patient to the hospital because she has multiple injuries to her face and hands. The physician in charge has ordered a facial bone series and bilateral hand radiographs. You have prepared the room for her arrival. The examination is progressing well when suddenly the patient begins to speak loudly. She is apparently arguing with someone named Bill. Bill is not present in the room. She is becoming more and more agitated.

➤ Identify the Following

GOAL

OBSERVATIONS

OPTIONS AND CONSEQUENCES

➤ Selection of the Best Option

GOAL

To obtain the radiographs needed for the patient's examination.

OBSERVATIONS

The patient is becoming delusional and very angry.

OPTIONS AND CONSEQUENCES

Option 1
Get out of the room as soon as possible and call security.

Consequence
You will not be able to obtain the radiographs needed.

Option 2
Do not become involved with your patient's delusions. Speak calmly and clearly. Explain what is needed for her examination. Position yourself so that you are near the door. Do not allow her to block your exit.

Consequence
You may be able to continue your examination.

Option 3
Speak to your patient in a calm tone and tell her that Bill is sorry for what he did. Tell her that Bill is waiting for her in her room. Tell her what she wants to hear in order to get a successful examination.

Consequence
You might get the examination completed.

Case 2.12 The Patient in Trauma

➤ Prerequisites

Before attempting this case study, the student should be knowledgeable of[24,25]:

- Positioning cervical spines
- Patient care for the patient in trauma
- Coworker relationships

DESCRIPTION ➤➤ Your patient is a 25-year-old man who was injured while diving into a shallow swimming pool. He is very muscular and stocky. He is supine on a stretcher and sandbags are placed on the sides of his head. The doctor has ordered a cervical spine examination. With the patient in the supine position, you have taken a lateral image of the cervical spine using a horizontal central ray. This radiograph demonstrates five cervical vertebrae, C1 through C5. The radiographer with whom you are working has stated that the only way to demonstrate the last two vertebrae is to pull the patient's shoulders down. He quickly puts on a lead apron and gloves and announces that he is "just going to yank his shoulders down a bit." You do not feel comfortable with his announcement. What do you do?

➤ Identify the Following

GOAL

OBSERVATIONS

OPTIONS AND CONSEQUENCES

➤ Selection of the Best Option

GOAL

To demonstrate all seven of the cervical vertebrae.

OBSERVATIONS

The C6 through C7 vertebrae are not demonstrated.

OPTIONS AND CONSEQUENCES

Option 1

You might suggest that the shoulders be pulled down as slowly and gently as possible.

Consequence

Pulling down gently on the shoulders minimizes the risk of further neck injury to the patient.

Option 2

Suggest placing a sheet or straps under the patient's heels. Ask the patient to hold the ends of the sheet and slowly work his hands down the sheet as far as they can go. If the patient experiences pain, tell him to stop.

Consequence

This procedure would probably allow the C6 through C7 vertebrae to be demonstrated with minimal injury to the patient.

Option 3

Take another radiograph of the patient's lower cervical region using the "swimmer's" technique.

Consequence

There will be distortion.

Case 2.13 The Paraplegic Patient

➤ Prerequisites

Before attempting this case study, the student should be knowledgeable of[26,27]:

- Patient care

DESCRIPTION ➤➤ Your patient is a 67-year-old male paraplegic who is scheduled for an intravenous urography (IVU) examination. You have prepared the room and brought him into the room. You have decided to change the patient into hospital clothes while he is on the x-ray table. The stationary x-ray table is higher than his wheelchair and it cannot be adjusted. What will you do?

➤ Identify the Following

GOAL

OBSERVATIONS

OPTIONS AND CONSEQUENCES

➤ Selection of the Best Option

GOAL

To move the patient onto the x-ray table and perform the IVU examination.

OBSERVATIONS

The patient is a paraplegic and is in a wheelchair. The stationary x-ray table is much higher than his wheelchair and cannot be adjusted to a lower position.

OPTIONS AND CONSEQUENCES

Option 1

When you arrive in the room, you immediately call for help in lifting the patient.

Consequence

Available technologists will lift him out of the chair and onto the table.

Option 2

You ask the patient what is the best way for him to be moved onto the x-ray table. You also ask him if he has any other needs.

Consequence

The patient remains in control of his surroundings.

Option 3

You locate the patient hoist device and have it delivered to your room.

Consequence

The patient can be hoisted out of the chair and placed on the x-ray table.

Case 2.14 The Patient Who Refuses an Examination

➤ Prerequisites

Before attempting this case study, the student should be knowledgeable of[28]:

- Medical ethics and law
- The Patient's Bill of Rights[4]

DESCRIPTION ➤➤ It is lunchtime and you have had a very difficult day. Your last two patients required a great deal of forbearance. Your next patient is a 79-year-old woman who is scheduled for a barium enema examination. You know that this examination is going to be extremely difficult to perform because you have read the patient's clinical history, which states that she has rectal bleeding. She arrived in the department via stretcher. She has just had a sigmoidoscopy and appears to be very tired.

The patient has soiled herself, and you must clean her before you can even start the examination. You have to review her chart to make certain that the examination has been ordered and that the consent form has been signed. You find all paperwork is in order.

As the patient moves onto the x-ray table, she complains about the hardness of the table and the temperature of the room. You bring warm blankets for the patient. You then gently explain the examination to her, telling her that you will do everything you can to make the examination as comfortable as possible. You explain to her the importance of holding the barium and she says that she just does not think she can. You obtain a scout radiograph of her abdomen. (A scout radiograph is the first radiograph taken before contrast media are used.) At this time, you tell her that the radiologist will soon be in the room to begin her examination. The patient begins to cry and asks, "Why are you doing this to me?" You explain that her doctor has ordered this examination. From reading her clinical data, you know that the patient has terminal cancer. You wonder why you're doing this to the poor woman. Why don't they just let her die in peace? You stand next to her and hold her hand. What is your next action?

➤ Identify the Following

GOAL

OBSERVATIONS

OPTIONS AND CONSEQUENCES

➤ Selection of the Best Option

GOAL

To give the patient the best care possible and to complete the examination.

OBSERVATIONS

The patient has terminal cancer and is questioning whether she needs this examination. You are very doubtful that the patient will be able to hold the barium.

OPTIONS AND CONSEQUENCES

Option 1

You explain to the patient that you have no idea why her doctor has ordered the examination. However, you are certain that there is a good reason. You then explain to her that it is entirely her choice whether to have the examination. You tell her that, if you were the patient, you would not have the procedure.

Consequence

The patient would probably refuse the examination.

Option 2

You explain to the patient that you know this is difficult for her. You also call her doctor and relay the doubts the patient has about this examination. Explain how tired the patient is and ask him if the examination can be performed at another time. You also ask the doctor to please speak with the patient.

Consequence

Chances are that the examination will be postponed until another time. This will give the patient time to speak with her doctor regarding any concerns she may have.

Option 3

You allay her concerns about the difficulty she may have with the procedure. You tell her that her doctor wants her to have the test and that he would be disappointed if she refused it.

Consequence

She will probably have the examination.

Case 2.15 The Patient with Alzheimer's Disease

➤ Prerequisites

Before attempting this case study, the student should be knowledgeable of[29]:

- The nature of Alzheimer's disease
- Medical ethics and law
- The Patient's Bill of Rights

DESCRIPTION ➤➤ Your patient is a 71-year-old man suffering from Alzheimer's disease. He has been scheduled for a radiograph of the chest. He has dyspnea and is in a wheelchair with an IV pole. His physician believes he may have pneumonia. As you bring the patient into the radiography room, he begins screaming and tries to get out of the chair. You speak calmly to him and explain that he is about to have a radiograph of his chest. You explain to him that it will not hurt and you will take the radiographs with him sitting in the chair. He seems to understand.

You have placed a cassette behind his back and positioned him for his chest radiograph. As you turn the x-ray tube toward the patient, he once again begins to scream. He leans forward and the cassette crashes to the floor. This increases his anxiety and he jumps out of the chair. The IV pole crashes to the floor. What do you do?

➤ Identify the Following

GOAL

OBSERVATIONS

OPTIONS AND CONSEQUENCES

➤ Selection of the Best Option

GOAL

To complete the chest examination.

OBSERVATIONS

The patient is in a wheelchair, suffering from Alzheimer's disease and possibly pneumonia. He is agitated.

OPTIONS AND CONSEQUENCES

Option 1

Restrain the patient against the back of the wheelchair. Slide the cassette between the restraint and the back of the chair.

Consequence

Completion of the examination.

Option 2

Request that a person familiar to the patient help you. Have that person stay with the patient while you prepare to make the exposure. Have the other person speak calmly to the patient and explain what is happening.

Consequence

Completion of the examination.

Option 3

Call the patient's nurse and request that the patient be medicated.

Consequence

The patient may not be able to take in a deep breath.

Case 2.16 Soft Tissue

➤ Prerequisites

Before attempting this case study, the student should be knowledgeable of[30–33]:

- Positioning
- Exposure technique
- Standard Precautions

DESCRIPTION ➤➤ You are working in the ED. Your patient is a 57-year-old man who was wounded by buckshot in the abdomen 2 months ago. He claims that he removed the buckshot pellets. He has a high temperature, swollen abdomen, and drainage from an open sore on his abdomen. The drainage has a strong, pungent odor. He has been examined by the ED physician, who has ordered a routine abdomen film to demonstrate foreign bodies, as well as another radiograph to demonstrate the area of abscess. The physician would like a radiograph profiling the soft tissue area around the abscessed region of the patient's abdomen. How should you proceed?

➤ Identify the Following

GOAL

OBSERVATIONS

OPTIONS AND CONSEQUENCES

➤ Selection of the Best Option

GOAL

Take an AP projection of the abdomen and another radiograph that "skims" the abscessed area.

OBSERVATIONS

The abscessed area is swollen and oozing what appears to be pus.

OPTIONS AND CONSEQUENCES

Option 1

Using Standard Precautions, take an AP projection of the abdomen using a standard exposure technique. Position the patient in a lateral position and rotate him posteriorly so that the abscessed area will be profiled.

Consequence

The AP abdomen will demonstrate metallic foreign bodies. The tangential projection will demonstrate the abscessed area.

Option 2

Using Standard Precautions, take an AP projection of the abdomen using an automatic exposure control (AEC) device. Position the patient in a lateral position, then rotate the patient posteriorly so that the abscessed area will be profiled. Use the AEC for this as well.

Consequence

The AP abdomen will demonstrate metallic foreign bodies. The tangential image may demonstrate soft tissue areas.

Case 2.17 Trauma Exposure Techniques

➤ **Prerequisites**

Before attempting this case study, the student should be knowledgeable of[34]:

- Trauma exposure techniques
- Pediatric radiography

DESCRIPTION ➤➤ You are working in the trauma center. Your patient is a 12-year-old girl who has been hit by a car. The physician has requested the following examinations:

Skull series
Chest
Abdomen
Pelvis
Bilateral femurs
Right elbow
Right forearm

You have obtained the equipment you will need and have determined the order in which you will x-ray the patient. You notice that the technique chart for pediatric patients is missing. The only technique chart that you have is for adult patients. How do you proceed?

➤ **Identify the Following**

GOAL

OBSERVATIONS

OPTIONS AND CONSEQUENCES

➤ Selection of the Best Option

GOAL

To obtain diagnostically acceptable radiographic images.

OBSERVATIONS

The technique chart that you have is for adults.

OPTIONS AND CONSEQUENCES

Option 1

Keep calm. You decide to use the same technical factors as you would on an adult, except that you will decrease the kVp by 15 percent for all of the exposures.

Consequence

This option may work.

Option 2

Keep calm. You obtain exposure techniques from another unit and attempt to use them.

Consequence

This option may work.

Option 3

Keep calm. Quickly observe the size of the patient. Compare the size of an adult's anatomical parts to the child's (e.g., the wrist of an adult might be the size of the child's elbow or forearm).

Consequence

This option may work.

Case 2.18 High-kVp Techniques in Gastrointestinal Examinations

➤ Prerequisites

Before attempting this case study, the student should be knowledgeable of[35]:

- GI positioning and procedures
- High-kVp techniques

DESCRIPTION ➤➤ Your patient is scheduled for a GI series. You have prepared the x-ray room for the examination. You have measured the patient for the scout film. Using the exposure technique chart, you have located a technique for a 22-cm abdomen. This exposure technique calls for the following: 10 mAs @ 80 kVp. You have shown the radiograph to the radiologist. On viewing the radiograph, he has requested a high-kVp technique. How do you proceed?

➤ Identify the Following

GOAL

OBSERVATIONS

OPTIONS AND CONSEQUENCES

➤ Selection of the Best Option

GOAL

To obtain a GI series using a high-kVp technique.

OBSERVATIONS

The technique for the scout film of the abdomen was taken at 10 mAs, 80 kVp.

OPTIONS AND CONSEQUENCES

Option 1

Request that the examination be completed in a room with an AEC device that is in good operational order.

Consequence

This option requires moving the patient but would probably work.

Option 2

To maintain the density found on the scout radiograph, reduce the mAs by a factor of ½ and increase the kVp by 15 percent. Your target range should be approximately 100 to 110 kVp. Keep in mind that you want the shortest possible exposure time.

Consequence

This option requires taking additional time to calculate the technique.

Option 3

Increase the kVp by 10 percent and decrease the exposure time station by one step.

Consequence

This option may work.

Case 2.19 Manual versus Automatic Exposure Techniques

➤ Prerequisites

Before attempting this case study, the student should be knowledgeable of[36–38]:

- AEC devices
- Manual exposure techniques
- GI anatomy

DESCRIPTION ➤➤ Your patient is a 65-year-old woman who had a barium enema examination 2 days ago. Today she is scheduled for a UGI series. As you evaluate the patient, you notice that she is extremely obese. You are uncertain if you should set a manual exposure technique or use the automatic exposure control device. You are also uncertain if you should use a rare earth screen. After careful thought, you decide to proceed as follows.

➤ Identify the Following

GOAL

OBSERVATIONS

OPTIONS AND CONSEQUENCES

➤ Selection of the Best Option

GOAL

To produce a diagnostically acceptable radiograph.

OBSERVATIONS

The patient had a barium enema examination 2 days ago. You have the option of using the AEC device or selecting a manual exposure.

OPTIONS AND CONSEQUENCES

Option 1

You elect to use the AEC device. You feel that this will take the guesswork out of how much exposure to use.

Consequence

If you are familiar with the AEC device in use, this may work.

Option 2

You decide to manually select the exposure factors. You feel that with careful planning, you will have more control over the radiographic image.

Consequence

Proper manual exposure techniques will produce diagnostically acceptable radiographs.

Option 3

You elect to use the AEC device and rare earth cassettes.

Consequence

Assuming familiarity with the AEC device and adjusting for the changes required by a rare earth system, this technique may produce diagnostically acceptable radiographs.

Case 2.20 Multiproblematic: The Pediatric Patient in Trauma

➤ Prerequisites

Before attempting this case study, the student should be knowledgeable of[39]:

- Pediatric radiography
- Positioning in trauma

DESCRIPTION ➤➤ Your patient is a 6-year-old girl named Emily. She has fallen from a tree house and injured her arm. She is sitting on a stretcher with a pillow under her elbow. Her mother is standing next to her and appears to be pregnant. The child is very anxious. Although Emily has been medicated, she is still very upset. The mother is comforting the child, but the child is quickly becoming hysterical. You have just received a requisition to x-ray the child's right forearm. You have introduced yourself to Emily and her mother and have explained what you are going to do. The mother appears to be comfortable with the procedure. You tell Emily that you want to look at her arm. On inspection, you notice that the arm is not symmetrical. You doubt if she can turn the arm at all. You mentally begin to prepare your strategy. At this point, you leave Emily and her mother and prepare the room for the examination.

The room has been prepared. You bring both the parent and the child into the room. The mother immediately states that she is pregnant and that she cannot help. She tells you that you must give Emily a protective device. You calmly tell the mother that Emily will be shielded for the entire procedure. You explain that the amount of radiation used will be minimal. You show the mother the lap shield and tell Emily that this will be placed on her abdomen. As the mother prepares to leave the room, Emily screams, "I want youuuu!!!" The mother tells the child that she cannot stay but that the child must have the radiographs. The child looks at the equipment and screams as loud as she can. She is starting to hyperventilate. You begin to feel that this situation is out of control. What do you do to obtain the radiographs?

➤ Identify the Following

GOAL

OBSERVATIONS

OPTIONS AND CONSEQUENCES

➤ Selection of the Best Option

GOAL

To obtain the radiograph while addressing the special needs of the patient.

OBSERVATIONS

Emily is very anxious about the radiograph because she is afraid it will hurt, she is afraid that her arm is broken, and she is upset about her mother's leaving the room.

OPTIONS AND CONSEQUENCES

Option 1

In your dealings with Emily, be very stern. Ask the mother to leave the room and explain to Emily that she is going to have the radiographs.

Consequence

Emily may cooperate for the examination.

Option 2

Speak directly to Emily while you show both Emily and her mother the room. Tell Emily that her mother will leave the room with you but will be watching her in the control room.

Consequence

Emily may feel more secure but may still be upset.

Option 3

Ask the mother to wait outside. Explain the entire procedure to Emily and show Emily the x-ray machine. Demonstrate the light and the sound that the rotor makes when it is rotating.

Consequence

Emily may get more upset when her mother leaves the room, but she may cooperate.

DESCRIPTION ➤➤ There is an additional problem of actually obtaining diagnostically acceptable radiographs of Emily's obviously injured elbow.

➤ Identify the Following

GOAL

OBSERVATIONS

OPTIONS AND CONSEQUENCES

➤ Selection of the Best Option

GOAL

To obtain a radiographic examination of Emily's elbow.

OBSERVATIONS

The patient is sitting on a stretcher with her elbow on a pillow. Her arm is very asymmetrical. This is consistent with a fracture or a dislocation. You doubt that the patient will be able to move her arm. Even if she is able to move the arm, the motion will be extremely limited.

OPTIONS AND CONSEQUENCES

Option 1

You will have to get help positioning the patient. If a nurse or another health-care worker could gently lift Emily's arm, you would proceed as follows:

Pull the lead apron higher up onto her pelvis.

Place a large block sponge with a cassette on top under her forearm. Radiographs could then be taken.

Consequence

Successful attainment of the radiographs.

Option 2

Gently remove the pillow from under the patient's arm. Gently lower the back of the stretcher so the patient is placed in the supine position. Slowly abduct the arm from the shoulder. Place a lead shield across the patient's pelvis.

Gently lift the fractured arm and place a cassette under it. Gently rotate the arm in the supine position and use a sandbag to hold the hand in the supine position. Obtain a radiograph of the arm in this position. On completion, turn the central ray into the horizontal position and place the cassette alongside the forearm, next to the patient's side. Obtain a radiograph of the arm in the lateral position.

Consequence
Successful attainment of the radiographs.

Case 2.21 Multiproblematic: Barium Enema Examination for a Geriatric Patient

➤ Prerequisites

Before attempting this case study, the student should be knowledgeable of[40,41]:

- Barium enema examinations
- Geriatric patient management

DESCRIPTION ➤➤ Your patient is a frail 96-year-old woman scheduled for a barium enema examination. She came from a local nursing home and has arrived in your department via stretcher. You immediately recognize her. Last week, you performed a GI series on her. As you begin to introduce yourself, you realize that she is no longer the alert woman that you met last week. She is extremely tired and a bit confused.

As you prepare the room for her examination, you place a mattress on the table. You prepare the contrast for the examination and take a scout film of her abdomen.

The patient and room are ready for the examination. You are preparing to insert the enema tip when you suddenly realize that the patient is wearing the same exact hospital clothes that you put on her last week. You become upset over this. What do you do?

➤ Identify the Following

GOAL

OBSERVATIONS

OPTIONS AND CONSEQUENCES

➤ Selection of the Best Option

GOAL

Complete the patient's examination.

OBSERVATIONS

Your patient is wearing the same hospital clothes that you put on her 1 week ago.

OPTIONS AND CONSEQUENCES

Option 1
Immediately call the State Department of Health.

Consequence
This may cause a delay in the completion of the examination and possibly involve you in a potential controversy.

Option 2
Tell everyone with whom you are working about your discovery and let them know how angry you are.

Consequence
You will gather popular support for your cause but will inevitably delay the patient's examination.

Option 3
Continue with the examination before discussing this with anyone. Complete the examination and then call your supervisor. Ask him or her what hospital policy is regarding this situation.

Consequence
You will have benefited the patient by expediting the examination, but you may now become involved in a controversy.

DESCRIPTION ➤➤ The examination has progressed to the fluoroscopic part of the examination. You are well into the procedure when suddenly the patient expels the barium. On the monitor you can see the barium pooling. The radiologist asks you to obtain what you can for radiographs. How do you proceed?

➤ Identify the Following

GOAL

OBSERVATIONS

OPTIONS AND CONSEQUENCES

➤ Selection of the Best Option

GOAL

To obtain the best radiographs that you can, quickly and efficiently, with as much of the pooled barium out of the way as possible.

OBSERVATIONS

The patient has expelled the barium and is lying in it.

OPTIONS AND CONSEQUENCES

Option 1

Work as quickly as you can. Remove the patient's soiled clothes. Clean up the pool of barium around her and take at least an AP radiograph.

Consequence

The longer it takes for you to clean her, the more barium will be expelled.

Option 2

Do not clean her immediately. Take AP and lateral radiographs and quickly show these to the radiologist.

Consequence

The images may be obscured by the puddle of barium.

Option 3

Explain to the patient that the examination will probably be repeated because she did not hold the enema.

Consequence

The patient will probably feel humiliated and anxious.

Case 2.22 Multiproblematic: The Pregnant Patient in Trauma

➤ Prerequisites

Before attempting this case study, the student should be knowledgeable of[42–45]:

- Radiation protection
- Positioning and technique setting skills

DESCRIPTION ➤➤ You have been called to the ED to x-ray a 27-year-old woman. According to the requisition, you are to obtain radiographs of her pelvis, bilateral femurs, and lower legs. You quickly set up the room and prepare for the examination. When the patient is brought into the room, she tells you that she is 3 months pregnant.

➤ Identify the Following

GOAL

OBSERVATIONS

OPTIONS AND CONSEQUENCES

➤ Selection of the Best Option

GOAL

To obtain radiographs of the patient's pelvis, bilateral femurs, and lower legs.

OBSERVATIONS

The patient is pregnant. You are uncertain if the ordering physician and nurse are aware of this.

OPTIONS AND CONSEQUENCES

Option 1

Because this is a trauma situation, you decide to take the radiographs. You can notify the physician that the patient is pregnant after the radiographs have been completed. You decide to complete the examination in the following order:

AP pelvis
AP right femur
AP right knee
AP right lower leg
AP left femur
AP left knee
AP left lower leg

Consequence

You will have introduced a radiation dosage into someone who is pregnant. However, this is a trauma situation.

Option 2

You notify the patient's attending physician of the pregnancy.

Consequence

The examination may be canceled or modified in some way by the physician.

Option 3

You tell the patient that you will x-ray her legs but will wait to x-ray her pelvis. You also tell her that when you are obtaining a radiograph of her legs, you can shield her pelvis from the radiation.

Consequence

If this option is acceptable in your department protocol, the patient may have to move onto the x-ray table twice.

DESCRIPTION ➤➤ You have informed the patient's physician that the patient is pregnant. He decides to consult with the patient's obstetrician and a radiologist before having you complete the examination. After consultation with the other physicians, the decision is made to complete the examination. How do you proceed?

➤ Identify the Following

GOAL

OBSERVATIONS

OPTIONS AND CONSEQUENCES

➤ Selection of the Best Option

GOAL

To complete the examination using appropriate radiation protection practices.

OBSERVATIONS

You will be able to shield the patient's pelvis while obtaining radiographs of the legs but not during the pelvis film.

OPTIONS AND CONSEQUENCES

Option 1

Measure the patient's pelvis and select appropriate exposure factors.

Consequence

The radiograph should be acceptable.

Option 2

Use a higher-kVp technique to reduce the mAs that you will need.

Consequence

You will decrease the exposure to the patient.

Option 3

Increase your screen speed. This should allow you to decrease your exposure factors by at least half.

Consequence

You will lose some detail but reduce the overall pelvic exposure.

Case 2.23 Multiproblematic: Lack of Radiation Protection in a Trauma Situation

➤ Prerequisites

Before attempting this case study, the student should be knowledgeable of[46,47]:

- Positioning of trauma patients
- Radiation protection

DESCRIPTION ➤➤ Your patient is a 45-year-old woman. According to the nurse, the patient is a carpenter who has fallen from a scaffold and injured her dorsal spine, lumbar spine, pelvis, and both femurs. She has arrived in the trauma center in the supine position. The physician in charge has requested that the patient not be moved. All radiographs are to be taken portable and with the patient in the supine position. The physician has ordered the following examinations:

Bilateral femurs
Dorsal spine
Lumbar spine
Pelvis

You have organized the examination in the following order:

Lateral dorsal spine (cross table)
Lateral lumbar spine (cross table)
AP dorsal spine
AP lumbar spine
AP pelvis
AP both femurs
Lateral pelvis
Right and left lateral femurs

You have obtained all of the equipment necessary for the patient's examination. The physician is very impatient for the radiographs and you feel pressured. You therefore quickly position the portable unit for the dorsal spine radiograph. You announce that you are about to take an exposure. The nurse in charge yells out that she does not have an apron. What do you do?

➤ Identify the Following

GOAL

OBSERVATIONS

OPTIONS AND CONSEQUENCES

➤ Selection of the Best Option

GOAL

To apply good radiation protection practice.

OBSERVATIONS

The nurse does not have an apron.

OPTIONS AND CONSEQUENCES

Option 1

Tell the nurse to stand behind you during the exposure.

Consequence

This could work as long as she is the same height or shorter than you.

Option 2

Tell the nurse that it is her responsibility to have an apron.

Consequence

This may cause more tension than is already present.

Option 3

Tell her to leave the room.

Consequence

It may or may not be possible for her to leave.

DESCRIPTION ➤➤ The images are viewed and the spine radiographs are interpreted as negative. The femurs are both fractured. The pelvis is also fractured. The next step is to produce lateral images of the pelvis and femurs. How do you proceed?

➤ Identify the Following

GOAL

OBSERVATIONS

OPTIONS AND CONSEQUENCES

➤ Selection of the Best Option

GOAL

To produce a lateral image of the pelvis and bilateral femurs.

OBSERVATIONS

The patient is not able to lift either leg to produce a lateral image of the hip area.

OPTIONS AND CONSEQUENCES

Option 1

Place a large grid so that it is in contact with the lateral aspect of the patient's pelvis. Direct the central ray horizontally through the patient's pelvis. This will demonstrate a lateral image of the pelvis. For the femurs, place a grid next to the medial aspect of each leg. Move the cassette as superiorly as possible into the patient's midline. Direct the central ray horizontally to the midpoint of the grid. Do this for both femurs. The upper hip areas can be demonstrated during surgery.

Consequence

You will demonstrate lateral images of the pelvis and most of the femoral areas.

Option 2

Place a large grid so that it is in contact with the lateral aspect of the patient's pelvis. Direct the central ray horizontally through the patient's pelvis. This will demonstrate a lateral image of the pelvis. For the femurs, place a grid next to the medial aspect of each femur. Move the cassette as superiorly as possible into the patient's midline. Direct the central ray horizontally to the midpoint of the grid. For the lateral image of the hip joint, position the patient for the inferosuperior projection of the femoral necks (Clements-Nakayama modification).[6] Make certain that the patient is as near to the edge of the table as possible. Place a grid so that it is in contact with the patient's lateral aspect of the pelvis. The lead strips must run horizontally, so that the grid is below the edge of the table. This will ensure that the entire upper femur will be included on the film. The top of the grid is angled 15 degrees posteriorly. The grid itself is also angled so that it is parallel with the femoral neck. The central ray is first placed horizontally and then angled posteriorly 15 degrees. It is directed to enter the medial-anterior aspect of the femur and exits the lateral superior border of the femur at the pelvis. This position should be used for both femurs.

Consequence
You will demonstrate lateral images of the pelvis. The mid-femoral to lower-femoral areas will also be demonstrated in a lateral image. The lateral image of the hips will be distorted.

Option 3
Place a large grid so that it is in contact with the lateral aspect of the patient's pelvis. Direct the central ray horizontally through the patient's pelvis. This will demonstrate a lateral image of the pelvis. For the femurs, place a grid next to the medial aspect of each femur. Move the cassette as superiorly as possible into the patient's midline. Direct the central ray horizontally to the midpoint of the grid. For the lateral image of the hip joint, gently oblique the patient's entire body. Place radiolucent sponges under the sides of the patient. Make certain that the entire femur is supported at all times. Direct the central ray perpendicular to the lowermost hip. Make certain to check this film before moving the patient into the opposite oblique position.

Consequence
You will demonstrate a lateral image of the pelvis. The lower femurs to mid-femurs will also be demonstrated in a lateral image. The hips will appear as an oblique image.

Case 2.24 Multiproblematic: The Pediatric Patient with Multiple Trauma

➤ Prerequisites

Before attempting this case study, the student should be knowledgeable of[48–51]:

- Positioning all parts of the body
- Skeletal anatomy
- Pediatric positioning, procedures, and pediatric care
- Organizing a trauma examination to improve efficiency

DESCRIPTION ➤➤ The patient is a 9-year-old boy who has been hit by a car. He is currently in the trauma room. The patient has sustained injuries to his pelvis and femoral areas. You have just been given a list of the areas that you are to x-ray. They are:

Pelvis
Chest
Abdomen
Bilateral femurs

You decide that the most efficient order in which to obtain these radiographs is as follows:

Chest
Abdomen
Pelvis
AP femurs
Lateral femurs with a horizontal central ray

You have obtained all of the equipment you will need and are just about to proceed with the examination when, on entering the trauma room, you suddenly realize that your patient is your neighbor. You are trying to focus on your work, but all you keep thinking about is what a nice kid he is. What should you do?

➤ Identify the Following

GOAL

OBSERVATIONS

OPTIONS AND CONSEQUENCES

➤ Selection of the Best Option

GOAL

To complete a successful examination.

OBSERVATIONS

This is a trauma situation. You know the patient and his family. You are upset.

OPTIONS AND CONSEQUENCES

Option 1

Call for help. Have another radiographer complete the case.

Consequence

This may be possible.

Option 2

Proceed with the examination. Keep focused.

Consequence

This may be possible.

DESCRIPTION ➤➤ The physician in charge has viewed the radiographs and finds that the patient's pelvis is fractured. The fracture has occurred at the area of the pubic and ischial rami. The nurse has catheterized the patient's urinary bladder and found that it has blood in it. A urologist has been called into the case and has ordered a cystogram of the urinary bladder. Instead of going to the cysto suite in surgery to perform the examination, he tells you that the procedure will be completed here. You are very uncertain of the exposure factors to use. The room that you are currently using does not have a moving grid, and you know that you will have to use a stationary one.

➤ Identify the Following

GOAL

OBSERVATIONS

OPTIONS AND CONSEQUENCES

➤ Selection of the Best Option

GOAL

To complete the cystogram as efficiently as possible.

OBSERVATIONS

Review the AP pelvis radiograph. Evaluate the technical factors used. Did the technique used demonstrate the bony structures and soft tissue? Picture the addition of contrast medium to the image with those factors. Would the film be too underexposed? Overexposed?

OPTIONS AND CONSEQUENCES

Option 1

Tell the urologist that you cannot perform the cystogram as a portable examination.

Consequence

The urologist will ask for someone who knows what he or she is doing to complete the examination.

Option 2

Position the patient for another AP pelvis examination, just as you did for the original examination, and increase your kVp to enhance the contrast medium.

Consequence

The increase in kVp will demonstrate an opaque, dilated bladder.

Case 2.25 Multiproblematic: Radiation Protection in Surgery and the Unreasonable Orthopedist

➤ Prerequisites

Before attempting this case study, the student should be knowledgeable of[52]:

- Radiography in the surgery suite
- Radiation protection
- Communicating with other health-care workers

DESCRIPTION ➤➤ You are working in surgery today, obtaining radiographs for a hip-pinning procedure of the right hip. You have brought the C-arm and monitors into the room before the start of the procedure. You have positioned the equipment with the orthopedic surgeon's preference in mind and hung the patient's initial radiographs (pelvis and hip) on the view boxes. The patient has been brought into the room and moved onto the surgery table, where you have positioned the patient and the C-arm. You are about to take a scout exposure of an AP projection of his hip. You announce that you are about to make an exposure. Suddenly the orthopedist screams that he does not have a lead shield. He immediately walks over to you and positions his face inches away from yours. He begins yelling at you that it was your responsibility to provide him with a lead apron or a lead-shielded wall. What should you do?

➤ Identify the Following

GOAL

OBSERVATIONS

OPTIONS AND CONSEQUENCES

➤ Selection of the Best Option

GOAL

To take an AP exposure of the hip.

OBSERVATIONS

The surgical suite is a sterile area with little or no inherent radiation protection facilities.

OPTIONS AND CONSEQUENCES

Option 1

Tell the doctor that you will get him an apron along with some mouthwash.

Consequence

Obtaining a lead apron for the doctor is a good idea; adding sarcasm is probably not.

Option 2

Tell him that it is the circulating nurse's responsibility.

Consequence

This will cause tension between the nurse and you.

Option 3

Tell the doctor you that will get him a lead apron.

Consequence

The procedure will continue.

The doctor has requested a C-arm image in both the AP and lateral projections. The AP projection is demonstrated very well. As you rotate the C-arm into the lateral position, you accidentally contaminate the sterile field. What should you do?

➤ Identify the Following

GOAL

OBSERVATIONS

OPTIONS AND CONSEQUENCES

➤ Selection of the Best Option

GOAL

To complete the examination.

OBSERVATIONS

You have just contaminated the sterile field. No one noticed, and only you are aware of the contamination.

OPTIONS AND CONSEQUENCES

Option 1
Say nothing.

Consequence
There may be no contamination.

Option 2
Tell the circulating nurse.

Consequence
The doctor will probably yell at you again.

AUTHOR'S OPINIONS

Case 2.1

Because your lateral images were acceptable, you should formulate a plan based on what is demonstrated on those images. You should know that on a correctly positioned reverse PA skull, the petrous ridges fill the orbits. To have the petrous ridges projected in the middle of the orbits, you would need to use a caudally angled central ray. The question is: How much of an angle? A useful trick is to picture two parallel lines: one running from the superior end of the orbit through the superior portion of the ear and the other running from the inferior end of the orbit through the inferior portion of the ear. The petrous portion of the temporal bone will lie within the area defined by these two lines. If you direct the central ray along this corridor, you will project the petrous ridge within the orbits.

For this reason, the best solution is Option 2. The consequences of Option 1 are simply not acceptable. Failing to attempt to obtain the best possible study does the patient no good. The patient is entitled to the best study that you can obtain under the circumstances. Nothing less is acceptable.

Case 2.2

Option 3 is the best solution. Obtaining radiographs of the hands and fingers in the supine position allows demonstration of both the metacarpal areas and the phalanges, provided that two exposures are used.

Obtaining radiographs of the hand in the AP oblique projection, Norgaard method (ball-catcher position), is also an excellent idea. This projection uses the natural position of the hand to demonstrate the joint spaces. This projection also requires that the central ray be directed between the two hands. This allows the divergence of the central ray to best demonstrate all of the joint spaces. The best analogy that I can give is that of an umbrella. If the main shaft of the umbrella is the midpoint of the central ray, this part would be perpendicular to the cassette. The spokes of the umbrella represent the natural divergence of the beam. When the hand is placed so that it is cupped (ball-catcher position), it allows the natural divergence of the central ray to demonstrate the joint spaces. The angle of the hand, along with the divergence of the central ray, demonstrates the joint spaces as well as the metacarpal heads.

Option 1 would produce an image that is distorted. In all likelihood, the metacarpal area would be demonstrated, but the phalanges would be curled onto themselves, and superimposition of these structures could take place. This distortion could hide important information. With the patient's history of rheumatoid arthritis, demonstrating the joint spaces is of the utmost importance.

Case 2.3

The best solution is Option 2 because the goal is to take diagnostically acceptable radiographs in the fastest and most efficient manner possible with the least patient discomfort. Clearly, the radiographer in the second option has chosen a very efficient sequence. All of the AP projections are taken first, starting with a high-priority examination (the chest), followed by the abdomen and lumbar examinations. The second half of the examination consists of the lateral radiographs. Once again, the radiographer starts from the most critical area. Keep in mind that during trauma situations, your prioritized list may suddenly change because of the patient's condition. However, the fact that you approached the case with a prioritized sequence means that you see the importance of working quickly and efficiently, keeping the patient's comfort in mind.

Case 2.4

Because of the patient's size, there is likely to be significant obstruction of bony detail if the radiographs are taken in an erect position. Also, an older female patient most often has a significant amount of bone demineralization. With this in mind, increasing the exposure factors, particularly the kVp, will not allow visualization of bone detail. It will only result in more graying of the image. This is because of the lack of calcium within the bones, rendering them more radiolucent.

For these reasons, the best solution is Option 1.

Case 2.5

The best solution is Option 2. With the patient placed in an LPO position, the fundic portion of the stomach is filled with barium. Because of gravity, the duodenum and pyloris will not be filled with barium. In the RAO position, the stomach empties very quickly. This is especially true of patients who have hypermotility of the GI tract. It may also be a good idea to take two RAO images of the stomach. These should be taken consecutively. This will demonstrate the changes that the stomach undergoes within seconds.

While Option 3 may be viable from a diagnostic standpoint, please keep in mind that it is the radiologist's, not the radiographer's, responsibility to change the type of contrast medium that is used for a study. It should also be noted that iodinated water-soluble contrast medium will actually stimulate peristalsis, thus defeating the purpose for the change from barium.

Case 2.6

Option 2 is the best choice. Although you acted in the best interests of the patient in Option 1, the taking of additional radiographs without the consent of a physician clearly violates the radiographer's "scope of practice." The option of additional radiographs is the physician's.

Case 2.7

The best solution is Option 2 because it is proactive rather than reactive. Option 3 may also be acceptable; the fact that you are a student does not mean that you do not know what you are doing. Speak to the physician. Ask him questions as necessary and do not be intimidated. For you to do your job successfully, you will need information from the physician. Once you know the approximate location of the catheter, you can begin to zero in. Use the information that is available before x-ray exposure. Where is the C-arm intensifier located on the patient's chest? Is the catheter high in the chest or is it in the right atrium? Once fluoroscopy is on, position the intensifier over the patient's midchest area, then begin to fluoroscope. At this point, locate areas that you are familiar with such as the spine, heart, or aortic arch. Use these structures to guide you. Quickly determine the approximate area that you are radiographing. Then look again at the placement of the intensifier. You may have to move the C-arm toward you or away from you. This can be accomplished by using the location of the spine as a landmark. Left of the spine are the patient's heart and aortic knob. The ribs will appear closer together the higher up into the chest you move. The ribs in the lower chest will appear thicker and set wider apart. Use these landmarks as guidelines.

Once you have located the area and the physician has requested that fluoroscopy be terminated, do not swing the intensifier out of the way. Instead, use the extension lock and move the intensifier back toward you. When fluoroscopy is requested again, simply extend the intensifier over the patient. Remember that even the most experienced radiographers have limitations. Keep focused on what you are doing and do not get frustrated, which can cause you to lose your concentration and confidence.

Case 2.8

Option 1 is the best solution. Discussing a confidential issue is against the Code of Ethics of Radiographers. We are also responsible for our actions, especially actions that could lead to a breach of confidentiality. Although you are not planning to discuss this case with anyone, you are aware that the patient came into the ED of the hospital in which she works. Information regarding her condition will certainly be available to a host of people. Taking all possible steps to ensure the patient's confidentiality minimizes that risk. However, Option 2 is almost equally valid. Protocols are established to ensure that breaches of confidentiality are minimized, while guaranteeing prompt, efficient patient care.

You have a responsibility to protect the information that the patient has given you. There are a few possible areas of concern, the first involving what you enter into the radiology computer system. Make certain that your information is accurate, but also be careful what you write. Accuracy and care should be used for all patient records. The other potential concern is that the radiographer working with you might see the radiographs and/or paperwork. If the other radiographer raises the issues, emphasize professionalism.

Case 2.9

Option 2 is the best solution. With this option, all attempts were made to produce the best radiographic image. Keep in mind that the amount of cephalic angulation will be determined by the degree of the patient's kyphosis. With this method, you are attempting to "lift up the chin with the central ray." If there is significant distortion on the cephalic-angled radiograph, obtain a second radiograph of the midchest area with the central ray directed perpendicularly. The radiograph with the cephalic central ray will demonstrate the area under the chin and the perpendicular central ray radiograph will demonstrate the main portion of the patient's chest. Submit both radiographs with an explanation.

Case 2.10

Option 2 is the better choice. The patient is having difficulty breathing, which is commonly seen with croup. With these symptoms, it is desirable to include the neck area on the radiograph to demonstrate the airway. For the lateral radiograph, it might be best to have the patient bring her arms behind her back (Pancoast Lateral). This will allow demonstration of the airway as well.

Case 2.11

The best solution is probably Option 2. However, it may be wise to alert the patient's nurse that the patient is becoming agitated. Keep in mind that you should position yourself between the patient and the door. This will allow you to have a quick exit, should the need arise. It is also a good idea to approach your patient from the side. Keep your conversation with the patient simple, and do not touch her until she has given you permission to do so. Option 3 should be avoided because it feeds the patient's delusions. She may become extremely upset when she discovers that you have lied to her.

Case 2.12

All three are good options. I am most comfortable with Option 2. By asking the patient to move his hands slowly down the sheet, you will cause the least amount of injury to the patient. If the patient is in pain (arm, neck, shoulder), he will be unable to perform this maneuver. On the other hand, having another radiographer apply gentle, even traction on the arms could possibly have the same result. This should be attempted only if the patient's physician gives permission.

Another technique that can be used is taking the exposure during complete expiration and having the patient relax his shoulders. The "swimmer's" method, also known as the Lateral projection, and the Twining method are other options. The Twining method requires the use of a grid and the ability of the patient to lift one arm up and over the head.

Case 2.13

Options 2 and 3 are viable solutions. However, did you notice that there is another problem in this scenario? It involves having the patient changed into hospital clothes.

It is always best to communicate with the patient before acting. This can be accomplished by first explaining the examination and asking the patient what he or she needs. The patient's spouse or companion may be in the waiting room, and the patient might feel more comfortable having this person's help. If this is not possible, then you should help the patient change into hospital clothes. This would require maintaining the patient's privacy and dignity as much as possible.

As far as moving the patient onto the table, ask the patient. Option 1 does not take the patient's desires into account. Keep in mind that requesting lifting help may still be necessary, but asking the patient first eliminates having a group of people standing around your patient and perceiving him as a problem. You maintain the dignity of your patient when you ask him what he can do on his own. Option 3 allows the patient to be moved onto the table with little risk of injury to other technologists. It is important that the patient communicate with you what he feels is best for him and that he listen to you for your opinion.

Case 2.14

Option 2 is the best solution. The patient's needs are kept in focus. At no time should a radiographer tell a patient what he or she feels should be done if he or she were the patient, as suggested in Option 1. Obviously, the patient's doctor feels that a barium enema examination is needed. However, the patient deserves to make an informed decision regarding her care. It is very tempting to gently coax a patient into refusing, especially if you question the appropriateness of an examination. On the other hand, it is ethically wrong to manipulate a patient into completing an examination, as is suggested by Option 3. The role of the radiographer is to provide support and give the best care possible.

Case 2.15

Option 2 is the best option. If possible, have a person with whom the patient is familiar stay at the patient's side. Perform the examination during a time when there is a minimal waiting period. Patients with Alzheimer's disease often become confused and frightened by their surroundings.

Although Option 1 appears viable, keep in mind that physical restraints can be applied to a patient only with a physician's order. Option 3 should be contemplated only as a last resort. Again, this would require an order from the physician in charge of the case.

Case 2.16

Option 1 is the best choice. Option 2 suggests using an AEC device for the tangential image. This is not a good idea for two reasons. Close collimation will not be possible when using an AEC device. This may cause the exposure technique to be terminated before demonstration of a diagnostically acceptable abdomen.

Case 2.17

Option 3 is the best approach. In a situation like this, when you do not have the opportunity to use an accurate chart, this is probably the safest solution. This solution works best for extremities. For example, an adult's knee and lower leg are similar in size to a child's femur. An adult's wrist is similar in size to a child's elbow.

For the pelvis, the best approach is to compare the size of the pelvis to that of an adult. A child's pelvis is approximately half the size of that of a small adult. With this in mind, halving the mAs and slightly lowering the kVp would probably work. You do not want to lower the kVp too much. Higher kVp values allow a wider range of exposure latitude. Using a higher kVp also decreases the dose to the patient.

Regarding the skull, the mAs used for an adult are roughly the same as or just a little more than you would use for a child. It is a good idea to record the exposure factors that you used to have a reference point, if needed.

Keep in mind that children are *not* small adults and that their weight and bone density can vary widely from that of an adult. Another area to consider is that older adults may have osteoporosis, and this condition would require a lower kVp level. Always factor these differences into your technique.

Case 2.18

The preferred solution is Option 2. This requires that you increase your kVp by 15 percent and decrease your mAs by a factor of ½. Keep in mind that you should decrease the mA instead of the exposure time. Remember that you want the shortest possible exposure time to minimize motion artifacts on the film. Option 3 is not a good idea, despite the fact that many technologists use this as a rule of thumb. Exposure time stations are not the same in all radiographic units. Decreasing in increments (or "steps") could reduce your exposure time by ½, ¼, or less. This is obviously not a good habit to follow. Before you make an exposure, you must know exactly what the exposure is and how it will affect the finished radiograph.

Case 2.19

The best solution is Option 2. This gives the radiographer more control in producing an acceptable radiographic image. AEC systems are often thought to take the guesswork out of radiography. This is simply not true. Using an AEC device requires accurate positioning and chamber selection. It also requires the radiographer to select the kVp, mA, and backup time. It is imperative that the chamber be located under the area you are attempting to demonstrate. In a GI series, if the activated chamber is located under a large pool of barium, the exposure will continue until either the backup time has been met or the barium has been thoroughly exposed. Likewise, if the activated chamber is placed under the air-filled fundus of the stomach, the exposure will be terminated in a short period. The film will appear to be underexposed except for the air-filled fundus. In regard to backup time, it is important that you set the backup time to no more than 150 percent of the anticipated manual exposure.

Case 2.20

The best option is Option 2. If the mother is in the room with the patient as long as possible, the patient will feel more secure. The patient's mother will be able to give the child support while you do your work. Keep in mind that if the child becomes hysterical, it may be necessary to have the mother stay in the waiting room. If this occurs, you should get help in restraining the child.

Case 2.20 (Continuation)

The best solution is Option 1. Another health-care worker should lift the fractured arm. Mishandling a fracture can lead to more injuries. It is also important to remember that lifting should be kept to a minimum. With this in mind, the first thing that must be determined is who will be responsible for what. The radiographer taking the radiographs should be responsible for the overall direction. The radiographer should discuss with the other health-care provider what is needed before anything is attempted. The arm should be gently supported above and below the fracture site. The radiographer should immediately remove the pillow, place a lead apron across the patient's pelvis, place a large positioning block sponge on top of the lead apron for support, and finally, place a cassette on top of the sponge. Make certain that the edge of the sponge is flush with the edge of the arm. This will allow easy placement of the cassette for the lateral image. Do not rotate the arm; ask the patient to turn it. If this is not possible, do not force it. Once the modified AP/PA radiograph has been obtained, remove the cassette in the same organized manner. Leave the sponge and lead apron in place. A new cassette should be placed next to the lateral aspect of the forearm. The cassette should extend below the edge of the forearm and alongside the sponge. For both exposures, ask the patient to hold her breath. This will help to eliminate any motion caused by the sponge moving during respiration.

Case 2.21

Option 3 is the best solution. Enlisting the aid of a government agency or your colleagues to help correct an obvious wrong may seem like the best course of initial action, but it does little to benefit your patient. In fact, it will be detrimental to your patient by delaying her procedure. Following up on the situation after the examination is finished is the best course to take.

Case 2.21 (Continuation)

Options 1 and 2 are valid solutions. How fast you are able to clean the patient and obtain a radiograph will determine the best course of action. Remember that the goal is to take the radiographs as quickly as possible and have the soiled barium out of the way. You may be able to have someone help you clean the patient. Option 3 is simply not acceptable. Telling a patient that she has to have the examination again is not in our scope of practice. This is a decision that would be reached by the patient's physician and a radiologist.

Keep in mind that, although Options 1 and 2 are acceptable choices in this instance, planning to use a retention enema tip or an inflatable bed pan "donut" before even starting the examination would have been better. You must be able to make realistic assessments of your patient's abilities and plan accordingly.

Case 2.22

Option 2 is the only possible choice. A physician should be made aware of all medical information regarding a patient before radiographs are taken. Proceeding with the examination in any form without notifying the physician is simply not compliant with the need to keep radiation as low as reasonably achievable (ALARA).

Case 2.22 (Continuation)

All three options should be considered, either singly or in combination. Using a faster screen will definitely reduce the overall exposure to the patient. Increasing the kVp slightly and decreasing the mAs will maintain density and also reduce exposure to the patient.

Case 2.23

The best option is to have the nurse leave the room. If this is not possible, have her stand behind you. You, of course, should be wearing a lead apron. It is the responsibility of the radiographer to provide radiation protection for other health-care workers.

Case 2.23 (Continuation)

The best solution is Option 2. Option 1 does not address the fact that the hip areas are not demonstrated. Option 3 suggests that the patient be turned into oblique positions. This would not be possible because of the fractures. Using this option would cause the patient considerable pain, as well as possible vascular damage. Option 2 suggests using the inferosuperior projection of the femoral necks (Clements-Nakayama modification position). This will demonstrate the hip joints with distortion, but it is still the best option considering the status of the patient.

Case 2.24

This is a very difficult situation. The best option is to have someone else perform the examination. This is true for two reasons. The first is that because of the upsetting nature of this situation, you may not be able to remove yourself from the situation sufficiently to perform the examination to the best of your abilities. The second is the issue of confidentiality. The patient's mother is going to ask you a lot of questions, many of which you may not be able to handle in a professional manner.

Without a doubt, the best solution is to remove yourself from the case. If this is not possible, you must prepare for the task at hand, which is, of course, a timely, accurate radiographic examination of the patient. Once you have completed the examination, you should give yourself the opportunity to do two things. The first is to express your sadness and anger in a private location, away from the turmoil of the ED. The darkroom may be the only place immediately available to you. The other is to prepare yourself for your encounter with your friend, the patient's mother. You should think through what your answers will be in regard to her questions. Keep in mind that the hospital chaplain may be of assistance to you.

Case 2.24 (Continuation)

The best answer is clearly Option 2. There is no reason why a portable cystogram cannot be performed this way. It may not be technically ideal, but it will demonstrate to the urologist the status of the patient's bladder. Although it is true that this image will be overexposed compared with the first image, remember that you are attempting to demonstrate different structures with this image (i.e., the patient's bladder, filled with contrast medium).

Case 2.25

The best option is Option 3. This allows the case to continue. Option 1 will cause difficulty between you and the physician, which in turn will cause difficulty for the patient. Option 2 is simply a lie. It is the radiographer's responsibility to provide adequate radiation protection for the surgical team.

Case 2.25 (Continuation)

Immediately tell the circulating nurse that you contaminated the field. Expect that the doctor will probably berate you again.

At the end of the case, speak with your supervisor. Explain what has occurred and document the occurrence. There is no reason why you should be spoken to in that manner. Follow this up with the doctor and explain to him that he has no right to address you in that manner and if he has a problem with your abilities, he should speak to your supervisor.

References

1. Ballinger, PW: Merrill's Atlas of Radiographic Positions and Radiologic Procedures, ed 8, Vol 2. Mosby, St. Louis, 1995, pp 227, 236–237, 242–245.
2. Ibid, pp 80–81.
3. Drafke, MW: Trauma in Mobile Radiography. F. A. Davis, Philadelphia, 1990, pp 184–185.
4. Norgaard, F: Earliest roentgenological changes in polyarthritis. Radiology 85:325–329, 1965.
5. Norgaard, F: Early roentgen changes in polyarthritis of the rheumatoid type. Radiology 92:299–303, 1969.
6. Stapczynski, JS: Fracture of the base of the little finger metacarpal: Importance of the "ball catcher" radiographic view. Emerg Med 9:145–149, 1991.
7. Drafke, op cit, pp 1–3.
8. Ballinger, op cit, p 412.
9. Bushong, SL: Radiologic Science for Technologists, ed 6. Mosby, St. Louis, 1997, pp 259–260.
10. Cullinan, AM, and Cullinan, JE: Producing Quality Radiographs, ed 2. Lippincott, Philadelphia, 1994, p 160.
11. Eisenberg, RL, and Dennis, CA: Comprehensive Radiographic Pathology, ed 2. Mosby, St. Louis, 1995, pp 69–70.
12. Ballinger, op cit, pp 105–108, 115.
13. Patton, TK, and Thibodeau, GA: Anatomy and Physiology, ed 3. Mosby, St. Louis, 1996. p 631.
14. Torres, LS: Basic Medical Techniques and Patient Care for Radiologic Technologists, ed 4. JB Lippincott, Philadelphia, 1993, pp 3–8, 30–32.
15. Kowalczyk, N, and Donnett, K: Integrated Patient Care for the Imaging Professional. Mosby, St. Louis, 1996, pp 144–145.
16. Patton and Thibodeau, op cit, p 626.
17. Torres, op cit, pp 3–6.
18. Wilson, BG: Ethics and Basic Law for Medical Imaging Professionals. F. A. Davis, Philadelphia, 1997, p 147.
19. Ballinger, op cit, pp 452–455.
20. Darling, DB: Radiography of Infants and Children. Charles C Thomas, Springfield, Ill, 1971.
21. Eisenberg and Dennis, op cit, p 33.
22. Pancoast, HK: Roentgenology of the thymus in infants and differential diagnoses of enlarged thymus and its treatment. Am J Med Sci, 180:745, 1930.
23. Torres, op cit, pp 124–125
24. Ballinger, op cit, pp 352–353.
25. Drafke, op cit, p 153.
26. Torres, op cit, pp 60–61.
27. Ibid, pp 6, 12–14.
28. Ibid, pp 58, 117
29. Anderson, KN, Anderson, LE, and Glanze, WD (eds): Mosby's Medical, Nursing, and Allied Health Dictionary, eds. Mosby, St. Louis, 1998, p 63.
30. Carlton, RR, and Adler, AM: Principles of Radiographic Imaging: An Art and a Science. Delmar, Albany, 1992, pp 507–508.
31. Selman, J: The Fundamentals of X-Ray and Radium Physics, ed 7. Charles C Thomas, Springfield, 1985, pp 358–361, 364–366.
32. Ballinger, op cit, p 509.
33. Cullinan and Cullinan, op cit, pp 137–141.

34. Ibid, pp 295–296.
35. Carlton and Adler, op cit, pp 505–507.
36. Cullinan and Cullinan, op cit, pp 21–24.
37. Curry, TS, III, Dowdey, JE, and Murray, RC: Christensen's Physics of Diagnostic Radiology, ed 4. Lea & Febiger, Philadelphia, 1990. p 59.
38. Ballinger, op cit, pp 5–7, 122–123.
39. Torres, op cit, pp 110–111.
40. Wilson, op cit, pp 108–109.
41. Torres, op cit, pp 3–6, 137–139.
42. Ballinger, op cit, p 32.
43. CFR ξ 35.20 ALARA Program, Nuclear Regulatory Commission.
44. Drafke, op cit, pp 220–221, 241–244.
45. Torres, op cit, pp 122–123.
46. Ballinger, op cit, pp 292–293.
47. Clements, RS, and Nakayama, HK: Radiographic Methods in Total Hip Arthroscopy. Radiol Technol 51:589–600, 1980.
48. Cullinan and Cullinan, op cit, pp 145–146.
49. Torres, op cit, pp 8, 12–16.
50. Ballinger, op cit, pp 183–188, 292–293.
51. Clements and Nakayama, op cit.
52. Torres, op cit, pp 57, 167–168, 177.

Bibliography

Anderson, KN, Anderson, LE, and Glanze, WD (eds): Mosby's Medical, Nursing, and Allied Health Dictionary, ed 5. Mosby, St. Louis, 1998.

Ballinger, PW: Merrill's Atlas of Radiographic Positions and Radiologic Procedures, ed 8. Mosby, St. Louis, Vols 1–3, 1995.

Bushong, S: Radiologic Science for Technologists, ed 6. Mosby, St. Louis, 1997.

Carlton, RR, and Adler, AM: Principles of Radiographic Imaging: An Art and a Science. Delmar, Albany, 1992, pp 507–508.

CFR ξ 35.20 ALARA Program, Nuclear Regulatory Commission.

Clements, RS, and Nakayama, HK: Radiographic methods in total hip arthroscopy. Radiologic Technology 51:589–600, 1980.

Cullinan, AM, and Cullinan, JE: Producing Quality Radiographs, ed 2. Lippincott, Philadelphia, 1994.

Curry, TS, III, Dowdey, JE, and Murray, RC: Christensen's Physics of Diagnostic Radiology, ed 4. Lea & Febiger, Philadelphia, 1990, p 59.

Darling, DB: Radiography of Infants and Children. Charles C Thomas, Springfield, Ill, 1971.

Drafke, MW: Trauma in Mobile Radiography. F. A. Davis, Philadelphia, 1990.

Eisenberg, RL, and Dennis, CA: Comprehensive Radiographic Pathology, ed 2. Mosby, St. Louis, 1995.

Kowalczyk, N, and Donnett, K: Integrated Patient Care for the Imaging Professional. Mosby, St. Louis, 1996, pp 144–145.

Norgaard, F: Earliest roentgenological changes in polyarthritis. Radiology 85:325–329, 1965.

Norgaard, F: Early roentgen changes in polyarthritis of the rheumatioid type. Radiology 92: 299–303, 1969.

Pancoast, HK: Roentgenology of the thymus in infants and differential diagnoses of enlarged thymus and its treatment. Am J Med Sci 180:745, 1930.

Patton, TK, and Thibodeau, GA: Anatomy and Physiology, ed 3. Mosby, St. Louis, 1996.

Selman, J: The Fundamentals of X-Ray and Radium Physics, ed 7. Charles C Thomas, Springfield, Ill, pp 358–361, 364–366.

Stapczynski, JS: Fracture of the base of the little finger metacarpal: Importance of the "ball catcher" radiographic view. J Emerg Med 9:145–149, 1991.

Torres, LS: Basic Medical Techniques and Patient Care for Radiologic Technologists, ed 4. JB Lippincott, Philadelphia, 1993.

Wilson, BG: Ethics and Basic Law for Medical Imaging Professionals. F. A. Davis, Philadelphia, 1997.

3

Performance Case Studies for the Laboratory

You will now apply the skills that you learned in Chapter 2 in a simulated clinical setting.

SUPPLIES

To properly perform the case studies that follow, you will need to use an x-ray room and have the following items, which should be obtained with your instructor's permission and returned when the case studies have been completed.

An assortment of cassettes with various screen speeds
Radiolucent positioning sponges
Grids and grid holders
Tape
Lead shields
Stretchers

Wheelchairs
Paper and pencils

HOW TO PERFORM SIMULATED CASE STUDIES

These case studies are designed to allow you to apply the information you have learned in the classroom in a setting that simulates reality as closely as possible. The scenarios will be set up by your instructor to allow you maximum input, participation, and performance. You should thoroughly enjoy participating in these sessions because you are allowed to be as innovative as you choose. In fact, more often than not, the instructors will learn different approaches from the students. This obviously benefits everyone involved, especially the patient.

These performance case studies directly support the outcome assessment goals and qualitative measurement goals set forth in *Standard Eleven* (Program Effectiveness/Outcomes) of the current *Joint Review Committee on Education in Radiologic Technology Standards for an Accredited Educational Program in Radiological Sciences.* At the end of each case study is a set of forms that are to be used to provide a qualitative and documented outcome for each student.

The evaluation forms that follow each case study are designed to be a quick and thorough means of assessing your performance. They are to be given to two instructors. One instructor evaluates the student who is performing the examination and another instructor evaluates the student who is setting the exposure factors. The assessment of your technical skills is concentrated in the following areas:

- Patient assessment
- Positioning
- Exposure factors
- Radiation protection (shielding, obtaining date of last menstrual period [LMP])
- Efficiency, leadership, and management

Patient Assessment

It is vital for students to develop the skills necessary to accurately assess the conditions of their patients. Although it is recognized that each health-care institution has its own established standards, protocols, and so on, the following is a suggestion for a general methodology for the assessment of patients:

Before performing the examination, the radiographer should:

- Obtain the patient's vital signs (vital signs are taken before, during, and after the examination).
- Obtain the patient history.
- Verify the correctness of the examination.

To ensure that you are providing the best possible care to your patients, an assessment similar to the following should be performed for every patient. Seven areas should be addressed during the patient assessment:

1. Mental status (alert, drowsy, unresponsive)
2. Respiration (labored, fast, shallow, hemoptysic)
3. Skin color (facial pallor, cyanosis, redness)
4. Bleeding (note bandaged areas, check for bleeding in the nose, mouth, and ears)

5. Sensory evaluation and pain (location of pain, intensity of pain, lack of sensation, tingling sensation, vision impairment, ringing in the ears [tinnitus])
6. Musculoskeletal integrity
7. Mobility (the patient's abilities)[1]

Positioning

Proper positioning is obviously important in producing an optimal radiograph. For each of the case studies, you will be assessed on your positioning skills as they relate to the case at hand. Your overall assessment will depend to a large degree on the accuracy and efficiency of your positioning skills and abilities.

Exposure Factors

Equally important to the production of an optimal radiograph is the proper use of exposure factors. Although it is recognized that there are wide variations in equipment capabilities from site to site, there are certain standards of exposure that can and should be maintained regardless of the equipment that is available. Each of the following studies has common optimal peak kilovolt (kVp) ranges for the major body regions. These values should be used as a guide only and adjusted according to your institution's requirements.

Radiation Protection

As a health-care professional using ionizing radiation, it is your duty to ensure that you are using proper radiation protection methods at *all* times. This applies to your patients as well as your fellow health-care workers. Although a complete discussion of radiation as low as reasonably achievable (ALARA) is beyond the scope of this book, all of your radiographs should exhibit evidence of collimation (which also improves your visibility of detail). Each institution has established protocols for patient shielding, but it is suggested that every patient having a radiographic examination be properly shielded. For women of childbearing age (this range is determined by the institution), a date for the patient's LMP should be obtained and her nonpregnant status verified.

Efficiency, Leadership, and Management

Not only are you assessed in terms of your technical skills, but you are also evaluated in the areas of organizational efficiency (i.e., how logical and efficient your approach is to the problem at hand) and leadership. The efficiency with which an examination is performed is fairly straightforward and can be easily evaluated in a clinical setting, but the concept of leadership is not easy to evaluate. However, a radiographer must exhibit leadership qualities to provide the best possible service and care to his or her patients.

Many excellent books are available on leadership and management, but the book that I have found most useful is one that we have in our family library, Roberts and Ross's *Make It So: Leadership Lessons from Star Trek: The Next Generation* (see Bibliography). Using the captain of the *Enterprise-D* as a role model for leadership in the 1990s, this book details the attributes of a true leader, such as Captain Jean-Luc Picard. The following attributes, which have proved to be of help in evaluating the leadership abilities of my students, should also prove helpful to you in establishing standards for yourself:

Focus—the ability to understand the "mission"
Urgency—what must be done and in what order
Initiative—searching for new ways around old problems
Competence—having the technical wherewithal to perform

Communication—being able to relay your message to the rest of the team
Politics—getting the job done without offending the team
Intellectual honesty—owning up to mistakes and limitations
Interdependence—working together toward a common goal
Resilience—seeing it through to the end

OBJECTIVES

On completing this section, the student will be able to:

Identify goals
Observe situations
List options
Select the best options
Demonstrate critical thinking skills within a specific time frame
Demonstrate organizational skills by performing exams in a logical order
Demonstrate leadership skills by instructing the assisting radiographer

DIRECTIONS

Participants

Two instructors—one monitors the positioning and procedure, and the other monitors the exposure factors.
Three students—one performs the examination and is "in charge" of the procedure, a second sets the exposure factors, and the third acts as the patient.
Class members—all class members observe.

An instructor reads the case study aloud to the class. The student who is performing the case study is given a specific time in which to perform the examination. A student plays the patient in the simulation. The student who is performing the examination determines the order in which the examinations are performed. That student is considered to be in charge of the examination. During the examination, the student radiographer will inform the student who is setting techniques of the cassette types and the routine that is to be followed. An instructor works with the student who is setting technique. The class observes the case study. At the end of the case study, the student in charge states why he or she chose the order in which the procedure was completed. The student who is selecting the exposure factors discusses why he or she chose the particular techniques and why. The class then discusses what might have been done differently and why.

Suggestions to the Student Who Is Performing the Case Study

- Assess your patient.
- Be aware of your patient's capabilities.
- Take charge.
- List the order in which the films are to be completed (using paper and pencil).
- Prioritize your examinations according to the needs of your patient.
- Obtain all equipment that you foresee being needed before beginning.
- Communicate effectively with your team.
- Do not waste time.

Suggestions to the Student Who Is Setting Exposure Factors for the Case Study

- Assess your patient.
- Communicate with the student in charge. Obtain the order in which films are to be completed.
- Write down the exposure factors that you have selected for each projection.
- Communicate effectively with your team.
- Be efficient.

SIMULATED CASES

In this chapter, read the prerequisites and description, then write your goal, observations, and the equipment you will need in the spaces provided. Use and attach extra paper if needed. Compare your answers to those suggested in the Author's Opinions following the case studies, then read the recommendations and exposure factors. Do this for each case study.

Case 3.1 Crushing Injury to the Chest

➤ Prerequisites

Before attempting this case study, the student should be knowledgeable of[2–4]:

- Trauma radiography, with the patient in the supine position
- Trauma radiography of chest and sternum

DESCRIPTION ➤➤ Your patient is a 24-year-old man who has been in an automobile accident and has received crushing injuries to his chest from the steering wheel. The patient has been intubated and is in the supine position. The following radiographic examinations have been ordered:

Chest
Sternum
Lateral
Oblique

You have 30 minutes to complete this examination.

➤ Goal

➤ Observations

➤ Equipment

You will need the following equipment:

Radiographic Procedure and Positioning Evaluation Form for the Student Performing the Examination (Student in Charge)

Student's Last Name ______

Student's First Name ______

Date ______

Equipment Necessary ______

	YES	NO	COMMENTS
Efficient organization of examination	☐	☐	
Demonstrates leadership	☐	☐	
Applicable shielding used	☐	☐	
Evidence of collimation	☐	☐	
Did the student: perform an acceptable patient assessment?	☐	☐	
interact with the patient appropriately?	☐	☐	

Acceptable?

Radiographic Projections	YES	NO	COMMENTS
	☐	☐	
	☐	☐	
	☐	☐	
	☐	☐	
	☐	☐	
	☐	☐	
	☐	☐	
	☐	☐	
	☐	☐	
	☐	☐	

GRADE ☐ PASS ☐ FAIL

Evaluator's Comments ______

Evaluator's Signature ______

Radiographic Procedure and Positioning Evaluation Form for the Student Setting Exposure Factors

Student's Last Name		Student's First Name		Date	

	YES	NO	COMMENTS
Demonstrates appropriate communication skills	☐	☐	
Demonstrates knowledge and applicable use of ALARA	☐	☐	
Demonstrates the ability to adjust exposure factors based on the patient's: age	☐	☐	
pathology	☐	☐	
condition	☐	☐	
Demonstrates the ability to adjust exposure factors due to changes in the following: SID	☐	☐	
film/screen combination	☐	☐	
grid ratio	☐	☐	

Acceptable?

Radiographic Projections	kVp	mAs	YES	NO	COMMENTS
	___	___	☐	☐	
	___	___	☐	☐	
	___	___	☐	☐	
	___	___	☐	☐	
	___	___	☐	☐	
	___	___	☐	☐	
	___	___	☐	☐	
	___	___	☐	☐	
	___	___	☐	☐	
	___	___	☐	☐	

GRADE ☐ **PASS** ☐ **FAIL**

Evaulator's Comments

Evaulator's Signature ______________________________

Case 3.2 Injury Caused by an Amusement Ride

➤ Prerequisites

Before attempting this case study, the student should be knowledgeable of[5–6]:

- Trauma radiography of the cervical, thoracic, and lumbar spine
- Radiation protection
- Exposure factors for these studies

DESCRIPTION ➤➤ Your patient is a 22-year-old woman who has been brought into the emergency department (ED) on a backboard. She was on a Ferris wheel ride at an amusement park when the seat broke and she fell approximately 6 feet, landing on her pelvis in the seated position. The patient states that she is very embarrassed and keeps giggling. She says, "My butt doesn't hurt, probably because of the padding." The following radiographic examinations have been ordered:

Cervical spine
- *Anteroposterior (AP)*
- *Both obliques*
- *Open-mouth odontoid*
- *Lateral*

Thoracic spine
- *AP*
- *Lateral*

Lumbar spine
- *AP*
- *Lateral*
- *Close collimated L5–S1 radiograph*

You have 40 minutes to complete this examination.

➤ Goal

➤ Observations

➤ Equipment

You will need the following equipment:

Radiographic Procedure and Positioning Evaluation Form for the Student Performing the Examination (Student in Charge)

Student's Last Name ______

Student's First Name ______

Date ______

Equipment Necessary ______

	YES	NO	COMMENTS
Efficient organization of examination	☐	☐	
Demonstrates leadership	☐	☐	
Applicable shielding used	☐	☐	
Evidence of collimation	☐	☐	
Did the student: perform an acceptable patient assessment?	☐	☐	
interact with the patient appropriately?	☐	☐	

Radiographic Projections	Acceptable? YES	NO	COMMENTS
	☐	☐	
	☐	☐	
	☐	☐	
	☐	☐	
	☐	☐	
	☐	☐	
	☐	☐	
	☐	☐	
	☐	☐	
	☐	☐	

GRADE ☐ PASS ☐ FAIL

Evaluator's Comments ______

Evaluator's Signature ______

Radiographic Procedure and Positioning Evaluation Form for the Student Setting Exposure Factors

Student's Last Name		Student's First Name		Date	

	YES	NO	COMMENTS
Demonstrates appropriate communication skills	☐	☐	
Demonstrates knowledge and applicable use of ALARA	☐	☐	
Demonstrates the ability to adjust exposure factors based on the patient's:			
age	☐	☐	
pathology	☐	☐	
condition	☐	☐	
Demonstrates the ability to adjust exposure factors due to changes in the following:			
SID	☐	☐	
film/screen combination	☐	☐	
grid ratio	☐	☐	

Radiographic Projections	kVp	mAs	Acceptable? YES	Acceptable? NO	COMMENTS
	___	___	☐	☐	
	___	___	☐	☐	
	___	___	☐	☐	
	___	___	☐	☐	
	___	___	☐	☐	
	___	___	☐	☐	
	___	___	☐	☐	
	___	___	☐	☐	
	___	___	☐	☐	
	___	___	☐	☐	

GRADE ☐ **PASS** ☐ **FAIL**

Evaulator's Comments

Evaulator's Signature ____________________

Case 3.3 Motorcycle Accident

➤ Prerequisites

Before attempting this case study, the student should be knowledgeable of[7,8]:

- Trauma radiography, with the patient in the supine position
- Trauma radiography of femur, hand, shoulder, humerus, and thoracic spine

DESCRIPTION ➤➤ Your patient is a 31-year-old man who is very muscular in build. While riding his motorcycle, he slammed on the brakes to avoid hitting a cat. His bike skidded into sand and "dumped" (motorcycle lingo for crashed), landing on top of him. His right side was injured. He is alert but understandably shaken. He was wearing a helmet, and according to the patient's nurse, a head injury is not suspected. The patient is supine and on a backboard. His clothes have been cut off and blood has saturated the sheets that he is on. His femur appears to be fractured. His shoulder is out of alignment and also possibly fractured. His hand is cut and has been loosely wrapped in gauze. The following films have been ordered:

Right femur
- *AP*
- *Lateral*

Right hand
- *PA*
- *Oblique*
- *Lateral*

Thoracic spine
- *AP*
- *Lateral*

Right shoulder
- *Internal rotation and external rotation*
- *Lateral*

You have 45 minutes to complete this study.

➤ Goal

➤ Observations

➤ Equipment

You will need the following equipment:

Radiographic Procedure and Positioning Evaluation Form for the Student Performing the Examination (Student in Charge)

Student's Last Name ______

Student's First Name ______

Date ______

Equipment Necessary ______

	YES	NO	COMMENTS
Efficient organization of examination	☐	☐	
Demonstrates leadership	☐	☐	
Applicable shielding used	☐	☐	
Evidence of collimation	☐	☐	
Did the student: perform an acceptable patient assessment?	☐	☐	
interact with the patient appropriately?	☐	☐	

Acceptable?

Radiographic Projections	YES	NO	COMMENTS
	☐	☐	
	☐	☐	
	☐	☐	
	☐	☐	
	☐	☐	
	☐	☐	
	☐	☐	
	☐	☐	
	☐	☐	
	☐	☐	

GRADE ☐ PASS ☐ FAIL

Evaluator's Comments ______

Evaluator's Signature ______

Radiographic Procedure and Positioning Evaluation Form for the Student Setting Exposure Factors

Student's Last Name		Student's First Name		Date	

	YES	NO	COMMENTS
Demonstrates appropriate communication skills	☐	☐	
Demonstrates knowledge and applicable use of ALARA	☐	☐	
Demonstrates the ability to adjust exposure factors based on the patient's:			
age	☐	☐	
pathology	☐	☐	
condition	☐	☐	
Demonstrates the ability to adjust exposure factors due to changes in the following:			
SID	☐	☐	
film/screen combination	☐	☐	
grid ratio	☐	☐	

Radiographic Projections	kVp	mAs	Acceptable? YES	NO	COMMENTS
	___	___	☐	☐	
	___	___	☐	☐	
	___	___	☐	☐	
	___	___	☐	☐	
	___	___	☐	☐	
	___	___	☐	☐	
	___	___	☐	☐	
	___	___	☐	☐	
	___	___	☐	☐	
	___	___	☐	☐	

GRADE ☐ **PASS** ☐ **FAIL**

Evaulator's Comments

Evaulator's Signature ______________________

Case 3.4 Fall from Roof

➤ Prerequisites

Before attempting this case study, the student should be knowledgeable of[9,10]:

- Trauma radiography with the patient in the supine position
- Trauma radiography of os calcis, lower leg, lumbosacral spine, chest, and elbow

DESCRIPTION ➤➤ Your patient is a 48-year-old woman who is currently in the psychiatric unit of the hospital. She apparently jumped approximately 15 feet off the roof of the hospital in an effort to escape. She had been missing for 2 hours, and it is now believed that she may have been lying on the roof of the hospital for that amount of time, apparently napping. Miraculously, she does not appear injured, except for a small scrape on her right elbow. She has since been sedated and is supine on the radiographic table. The physician in charge does not want her moved from the supine position and has requested that the following examinations be performed:

Bilateral os calcis
Right leg
Lumbosacral spine
Pelvis
Chest
Right elbow

You have 40 minutes to complete this study.

➤ Goal

➤ Observations

➤ Equipment

You will need the following equipment:

Radiographic Procedure and Positioning Evaluation Form for the Student Performing the Examination (Student in Charge)

Student's Last Name ____

Student's First Name ____

Date ____

Equipment Necessary ____

	YES	NO	COMMENTS
Efficient organization of examination	☐	☐	
Demonstrates leadership	☐	☐	
Applicable shielding used	☐	☐	
Evidence of collimation	☐	☐	
Did the student: perform an acceptable patient assessment?	☐	☐	
interact with the patient appropriately?	☐	☐	

Radiographic Projections	Acceptable? YES	NO	COMMENTS
	☐	☐	
	☐	☐	
	☐	☐	
	☐	☐	
	☐	☐	
	☐	☐	
	☐	☐	
	☐	☐	
	☐	☐	
	☐	☐	

GRADE ☐ PASS ☐ FAIL

Evaluator's Comments ____

Evaluator's Signature ____

Radiographic Procedure and Positioning Evaluation Form for the Student Setting Exposure Factors

Student's Last Name		**Student's First Name**		**Date**	

	YES	NO	COMMENTS
Demonstrates appropriate communication skills	☐	☐	
Demonstrates knowledge and applicable use of ALARA	☐	☐	
Demonstrates the ability to adjust exposure factors based on the patient's:			
age	☐	☐	
pathology	☐	☐	
condition	☐	☐	
Demonstrates the ability to adjust exposure factors due to changes in the following:			
SID	☐	☐	
film/screen combination	☐	☐	
grid ratio	☐	☐	

Radiographic Projections	kVp	mAs	Acceptable? YES	NO	**COMMENTS**
	____	____	☐	☐	
	____	____	☐	☐	
	____	____	☐	☐	
	____	____	☐	☐	
	____	____	☐	☐	
	____	____	☐	☐	
	____	____	☐	☐	
	____	____	☐	☐	
	____	____	☐	☐	
	____	____	☐	☐	

GRADE ☐ **PASS** ☐ **FAIL**

Evaulator's Comments

Evaulator's Signature ______________________________

Case 3.5 Electrical Shock with Burns and Trauma

➤ Prerequisites

Before attempting this case study, the student should be knowledgeable of [11,12]:

- Trauma radiography with the patient in the supine position
- Trauma radiography of scapula, ribs, and sternum

DESCRIPTION ➤➤ Your patient is a 46-year-old utility lineman who was working on the transformer on an electrical pole. According to a witness, a runaway truck hit the pole and the patient fell backward. In an effort to regain his balance, he accidentally grabbed two wires, received electrical current through his body, and apparently lost consciousness. He claims that he feels the most pain over both scapular areas. A witness who saw the incident states that the lineman struck his chest on the ladder. He has been admitted to the ED with electrocution burns on his chest. He has been given pain medication and is currently alert. The physician in charge has ordered:

Both scapulae
AP
Lateral
Sternum
RAO
Lateral
Bilateral ribs
AP below diaphragm
AP above diaphragm
Obliques

The patient is the supine position. The physician states that if the patient is able, he may turn very slightly. He may not sit.

You have 30 minutes to complete this examination.

➤ Goal

➤ Observations

➤ Equipment

You will need the following equipment:

Radiographic Procedure and Positioning Evaluation Form for the Student Performing the Examination (Student in Charge)

Student's Last Name ______

Student's First Name ______

Date ______

Equipment Necessary ______

	YES	NO	COMMENTS
Efficient organization of examination	☐	☐	
Demonstrates leadership	☐	☐	
Applicable shielding used	☐	☐	
Evidence of collimation	☐	☐	
Did the student: perform an acceptable patient assessment?	☐	☐	
interact with the patient appropriately?	☐	☐	

Acceptable?

Radiographic Projections	**YES**	**NO**	**COMMENTS**
	☐	☐	
	☐	☐	
	☐	☐	
	☐	☐	
	☐	☐	
	☐	☐	
	☐	☐	
	☐	☐	
	☐	☐	
	☐	☐	

GRADE ☐ PASS ☐ FAIL

Evaluator's Comments ______

Evaluator's Signature ______

Radiographic Procedure and Positioning Evaluation Form for the Student Setting Exposure Factors

Student's Last Name		Student's First Name		Date	

	YES	NO	COMMENTS
Demonstrates appropriate communication skills	☐	☐	
Demonstrates knowledge and applicable use of ALARA	☐	☐	
Demonstrates the ability to adjust exposure factors based on the patient's:			
age	☐	☐	
pathology	☐	☐	
condition	☐	☐	
Demonstrates the ability to adjust exposure factors due to changes in the following:			
SID	☐	☐	
film/screen combination	☐	☐	
grid ratio	☐	☐	

Radiographic Projections	kVp	mAs	Acceptable? YES	NO	COMMENTS
	___	___	☐	☐	
	___	___	☐	☐	
	___	___	☐	☐	
	___	___	☐	☐	
	___	___	☐	☐	
	___	___	☐	☐	
	___	___	☐	☐	
	___	___	☐	☐	
	___	___	☐	☐	
	___	___	☐	☐	

GRADE ☐ **PASS** ☐ **FAIL**

Evaulator's Comments

Evaulator's Signature ______________________________

Case 3.6 Fall from a Horse

➤ Prerequisites

Before attempting this case study, the student should be knowledgeable of[13,14]:

- Trauma radiography with the patient in the prone position
- Trauma radiography of sacroiliac joints, pelvis, sacrum, and coccyx

DESCRIPTION ➤➤ Your patient is a 45-year-old woman who fell from a horse and landed in a pile of horse manure. The odor in the examining room is very strong. The patient is in the prone position. The physician in charge has requested that the patient not be moved from this position and that he be allowed to position the patient for the oblique radiographs. The physician is extremely impatient. He has requested the following radiographic examinations:

Pelvis
  Posteroanterior (PA)
Lumbar spine
  PA
  Lateral
  Both obliques
Sacrum and coccyx
  PA sacrum
  PA coccyx
  Laterals of both
Sacroiliac (SI) joints
  PA axial
  Oblique SI joints

You have 45 minutes to complete this study.

➤ Goal

➤ Observations

➤ Equipment

You will need the following equipment:

Radiographic Procedure and Positioning Evaluation Form for the Student Performing the Examination (Student in Charge)

Student's Last Name ☐

Student's First Name ☐

Date ☐

Equipment Necessary ☐

	YES	NO	COMMENTS
Efficient organization of examination	☐	☐	
Demonstrates leadership	☐	☐	
Applicable shielding used	☐	☐	
Evidence of collimation	☐	☐	
Did the student:			
perform an acceptable patient assessment?	☐	☐	
interact with the patient appropriately?	☐	☐	

Radiographic Projections	Acceptable? YES	NO	COMMENTS
	☐	☐	
	☐	☐	
	☐	☐	
	☐	☐	
	☐	☐	
	☐	☐	
	☐	☐	
	☐	☐	
	☐	☐	
	☐	☐	

GRADE ☐ PASS ☐ FAIL

Evaluator's Comments

Evaluator's Signature ____________________

Radiographic Procedure and Positioning Evaluation Form for the Student Setting Exposure Factors

Student's Last Name		Student's First Name		Date	

	YES	NO	COMMENTS
Demonstrates appropriate communication skills	☐	☐	
Demonstrates knowledge and applicable use of ALARA	☐	☐	
Demonstrates the ability to adjust exposure factors based on the patient's:			
age	☐	☐	
pathology	☐	☐	
condition	☐	☐	
Demonstrates the ability to adjust exposure factors due to changes in the following:			
SID	☐	☐	
film/screen combination	☐	☐	
grid ratio	☐	☐	

Radiographic Projections	kVp	mAs	Acceptable? YES	NO	COMMENTS
	___	___	☐	☐	
	___	___	☐	☐	
	___	___	☐	☐	
	___	___	☐	☐	
	___	___	☐	☐	
	___	___	☐	☐	
	___	___	☐	☐	
	___	___	☐	☐	
	___	___	☐	☐	
	___	___	☐	☐	

GRADE ☐ **PASS** ☐ **FAIL**

Evaluator's Comments

Evaluator's Signature ______________________________

Case 3.7 Ambulatory Cervical Spine Examination

➤ Prerequisites

Before attempting this case study, the student should be knowledgeable of[15–17]:

- Radiography of the cervical spine in the seated position

DESCRIPTION ➤➤ Your patient is a 42-year-old man who walked into the ED, stating that he injured his neck while wrestling with his son and has had pain for 2 days. According to his radiograph requisition, a cervical spine has been ordered.

You bring the patient into the radiology room and introduce yourself. You perform your initial assessment of the patient by asking him what happened and where the pain is. You also ask him if he feels a tingling sensation in either arm. He states that he does not. He is very talkative and appears embarrassed that his 13-year-old son won the wrestling match. He states that, although he has had the pain for 2 days, he feels that the injury is due to his age and the fact that he is not in shape. It is obvious that he feels foolish for coming to the ED.

You have prepared the room for his examination and have explained the examination to the patient. You also tell him that you would like to have him hold sandbags for the examination. You ask him if he thinks he can. He states that he should be able to, but the fingertips on his right hand are numb. He states that he must have "slept in an awkward position." The following studies have been ordered:

Cervical spine
AP
Lateral
Odontoid projection
Both obliques

You have 30 minutes to complete this examination.

➤ Goal

➤ Observations

➤ Equipment

You will need the following equipment:

Radiographic Procedure and Positioning Evaluation Form for the Student Performing the Examination (Student in Charge)

Student's Last Name ______

Student's First Name ______

Date ______

Equipment Necessary ______

	YES	NO	COMMENTS
Efficient organization of examination	☐	☐	
Demonstrates leadership	☐	☐	
Applicable shielding used	☐	☐	
Evidence of collimation	☐	☐	
Did the student: perform an acceptable patient assessment?	☐	☐	
interact with the patient appropriately?	☐	☐	

Radiographic Projections	Acceptable? YES	NO	COMMENTS
	☐	☐	
	☐	☐	
	☐	☐	
	☐	☐	
	☐	☐	
	☐	☐	
	☐	☐	
	☐	☐	
	☐	☐	
	☐	☐	

GRADE ☐ PASS ☐ FAIL

Evaluator's Comments ______

Evaluator's Signature ______

Radiographic Procedure and Positioning Evaluation Form for the Student Setting Exposure Factors

Student's Last Name		Student's First Name		Date	

	YES	NO	COMMENTS
Demonstrates appropriate communication skills	☐	☐	
Demonstrates knowledge and applicable use of ALARA	☐	☐	
Demonstrates the ability to adjust exposure factors based on the patient's:			
age	☐	☐	
pathology	☐	☐	
condition	☐	☐	
Demonstrates the ability to adjust exposure factors due to changes in the following:			
SID	☐	☐	
film/screen combination	☐	☐	
grid ratio	☐	☐	

Radiographic Projections	kVp	mAs	Acceptable? YES	NO	COMMENTS
	____	____	☐	☐	
	____	____	☐	☐	
	____	____	☐	☐	
	____	____	☐	☐	
	____	____	☐	☐	
	____	____	☐	☐	
	____	____	☐	☐	
	____	____	☐	☐	
	____	____	☐	☐	
	____	____	☐	☐	

GRADE ☐ **PASS** ☐ **FAIL**

Evaulator's Comments

Evaulator's Signature ______________________________

Case 3.8 Fall on Ice

➤ Prerequisites

Before attempting this case study, the student should be knowledgeable of[18, 19]:

- Trauma radiography in the supine position
- Trauma radiography of the elbow, forearm, pelvis, and hip

DESCRIPTION ➤➤ Your patient is a 76-year-old woman who, according to her neighbor, fell on the ice while she was filling her bird feeder. She has been brought to the x-ray room in the supine position. She appears to be asthenic and kyphotic in body habitus. The physician has ordered the following radiographs:

Right elbow
AP
Lateral
Medial oblique
Lateral oblique
Right forearm
AP
Lateral
Pelvis
AP
Right hip
AP
Lateral

You introduce yourself to your patient and immediately notice that she is alert and does not seem to be in pain. In fact, she is talkative and very concerned that she was not able to fill the bird feeder. "Those birds count on me," she says. She suddenly begins to cry. "I can't believe that this has happened," she says. "I used to be an excellent ice skater." You notice that her right foot is laterally rotated and that the right leg is slightly shorter than the left. You also notice that her left elbow is bleeding and appears to be misshapen. You quickly surmise that she probably has a fracture of her right hip and right elbow.

You have 30 minutes to complete the procedure.

➤ Goal

➤ Observations

➤ Equipment

You will need the following equipment:

Radiographic Procedure and Positioning Evaluation Form for the Student Performing the Examination (Student in Charge)

Student's Last Name	
Student's First Name	
Date	

Equipment Necessary

	YES	NO	COMMENTS
Efficient organization of examination	☐	☐	
Demonstrates leadership	☐	☐	
Applicable shielding used	☐	☐	
Evidence of collimation	☐	☐	
Did the student: perform an acceptable patient assessment?	☐	☐	
interact with the patient appropriately?	☐	☐	

Acceptable?

Radiographic Projections	YES	NO	COMMENTS
	☐	☐	
	☐	☐	
	☐	☐	
	☐	☐	
	☐	☐	
	☐	☐	
	☐	☐	
	☐	☐	
	☐	☐	
	☐	☐	

GRADE ☐ PASS ☐ FAIL

Evaluator's Comments

Evaluator's Signature ______________________

Radiographic Procedure and Positioning Evaluation Form for the Student Setting Exposure Factors

Student's Last Name		Student's First Name		Date	

	YES	NO	COMMENTS
Demonstrates appropriate communication skills	☐	☐	
Demonstrates knowledge and applicable use of ALARA	☐	☐	
Demonstrates the ability to adjust exposure factors based on the patient's:			
age	☐	☐	
pathology	☐	☐	
condition	☐	☐	
Demonstrates the ability to adjust exposure factors due to changes in the following:			
SID	☐	☐	
film/screen combination	☐	☐	
grid ratio	☐	☐	

Radiographic Projections	kVp	mAs	Acceptable? YES	NO	COMMENTS
	___	___	☐	☐	
	___	___	☐	☐	
	___	___	☐	☐	
	___	___	☐	☐	
	___	___	☐	☐	
	___	___	☐	☐	
	___	___	☐	☐	
	___	___	☐	☐	
	___	___	☐	☐	
	___	___	☐	☐	

GRADE ☐ **PASS** ☐ **FAIL**

Evaulator's Comments

Evaulator's Signature ______________________

Case 3.9 Motor Vehicle Accident

➤ Prerequisites

Before attempting this case study, the student should be knowledgeable of[20, 21]:

- Trauma radiography in the supine position
- Trauma radiography of the abdomen, chest, lumbosacral spine, and skull

DESCRIPTION ➤➤ You have been alerted that a patient will be arriving in the trauma center within minutes. You have been given the following information: a 51-year-old man has been injured in an automobile accident. There are injuries to abdomen, skull, chest, and lumbar spine.

The patient arrives and is quickly assessed. He appears to have an abdominal injury. However, the nurse states that the patient has clear fluid coming out of his right ear. The patient is nonresponsive. An anesthesiologist has just intubated the patient. An IV is in the process of being started. The patient's abdomen appears to be very large in relation to his body. His condition is critical. The physician has ordered the following radiographic examinations:

Skull
AP (Caldwell)
AP axial (Towne method [also called Grashey method and Towne-Chamberlain method])
Lateral
Chest
AP
Lumbar spine
AP
Lateral
Abdomen
AP

You have 30 minutes to complete this examination.

➤ Goal

➤ Observations

➤ Equipment

You will need the following equipment:

Radiographic Procedure and Positioning Evaluation Form for the Student Performing the Examination (Student in Charge)

Student's Last Name ☐

Student's First Name ☐

Date ☐

Equipment Necessary ☐

	YES	NO	COMMENTS
Efficient organization of examination	☐	☐	
Demonstrates leadership	☐	☐	
Applicable shielding used	☐	☐	
Evidence of collimation	☐	☐	
Did the student:			
perform an acceptable patient assessment?	☐	☐	
interact with the patient appropriately?	☐	☐	

Acceptable?

Radiographic Projections	YES	NO	COMMENTS
	☐	☐	
	☐	☐	
	☐	☐	
	☐	☐	
	☐	☐	
	☐	☐	
	☐	☐	
	☐	☐	
	☐	☐	
	☐	☐	

GRADE ☐ PASS ☐ FAIL

Evaluator's Comments ☐

Evaluator's Signature ____________________

Radiographic Procedure and Positioning Evaluation Form for the Student Setting Exposure Factors

Student's Last Name		Student's First Name		Date	

	YES	NO	COMMENTS
Demonstrates appropriate communication skills	☐	☐	
Demonstrates knowledge and applicable use of ALARA	☐	☐	
Demonstrates the ability to adjust exposure factors based on the patient's:			
age	☐	☐	
pathology	☐	☐	
condition	☐	☐	
Demonstrates the ability to adjust exposure factors due to changes in the following:			
SID	☐	☐	
film/screen combination	☐	☐	
grid ratio	☐	☐	

Radiographic Projections	kVp	mAs	Acceptable? YES	NO	COMMENTS
	____	____	☐	☐	
	____	____	☐	☐	
	____	____	☐	☐	
	____	____	☐	☐	
	____	____	☐	☐	
	____	____	☐	☐	
	____	____	☐	☐	
	____	____	☐	☐	
	____	____	☐	☐	
	____	____	☐	☐	

GRADE ☐ **PASS** ☐ **FAIL**

Evaulator's Comments

Evaulator's Signature ____________________

Case 3.10 Blunt Trauma to the Face

➤ Prerequisites

Before attempting this case study, the student should be knowledgeable of[22–27]:

- Trauma radiography, with the patient in the supine position
- Trauma radiography of facial bones and skull

DESCRIPTION ➤➤ Your patient is a 49-year-old nonresponsive woman who has received blunt trauma to the face and skull during an assault. According to the patient's computer records, she is currently being treated for multiple myeloma. She is in the supine position. You have asked the patient's physician if a small sponge may be placed under the patient's head and if her neck may be turned slightly. The physician has agreed to both requests. The following examinations have been ordered:

Skull
AP axial projection (Towne method)
PA skull
Both laterals
Facial bones
Parietoacanthial projection (Water's method)
Lateral
Zygoma
Submentovertical (SMV)
Mandible
PA projection
Axiolateral oblique projection for the mandibular rami (bilateral)

You have 30 minutes to complete this examination.

➤ Goal

➤ Observations

➤ Equipment

You will need the following equipment:

Radiographic Procedure and Positioning Evaluation Form for the Student Performing the Examination (Student in Charge)

Student's Last Name ☐

Student's First Name ☐

Date ☐

Equipment Necessary ☐

	YES	NO	COMMENTS
Efficient organization of examination	☐	☐	
Demonstrates leadership	☐	☐	
Applicable shielding used	☐	☐	
Evidence of collimation	☐	☐	
Did the student: perform an acceptable patient assessment?	☐	☐	
interact with the patient appropriately?	☐	☐	

Acceptable?

Radiographic Projections	YES	NO	COMMENTS
	☐	☐	
	☐	☐	
	☐	☐	
	☐	☐	
	☐	☐	
	☐	☐	
	☐	☐	
	☐	☐	
	☐	☐	
	☐	☐	

GRADE ☐ PASS ☐ FAIL

Evaluator's Comments

Evaluator's Signature ____________________

Radiographic Procedure and Positioning Evaluation Form for the Student Setting Exposure Factors

Student's Last Name		Student's First Name		Date	

	YES	NO	COMMENTS
Demonstrates appropriate communication skills	☐	☐	
Demonstrates knowledge and applicable use of ALARA	☐	☐	
Demonstrates the ability to adjust exposure factors based on the patient's:			
age	☐	☐	
pathology	☐	☐	
condition	☐	☐	
Demonstrates the ability to adjust exposure factors due to changes in the following:			
SID	☐	☐	
film/screen combination	☐	☐	
grid ratio	☐	☐	

Acceptable?

Radiographic Projections	kVp	mAs	YES	NO	COMMENTS
	____	____	☐	☐	
	____	____	☐	☐	
	____	____	☐	☐	
	____	____	☐	☐	
	____	____	☐	☐	
	____	____	☐	☐	
	____	____	☐	☐	
	____	____	☐	☐	
	____	____	☐	☐	
	____	____	☐	☐	

GRADE ☐ **PASS** ☐ **FAIL**

Evaulator's Comments

Evaulator's Signature ______________________________

AUTHOR'S OPINIONS

Case 3.1

➤ Goal

To successfully complete the procedure in a satisfactory manner.

➤ Observations

The patient is intubated. This situation may require that the student take inspiration and expiration studies of the chest to demonstrate a pneumothorax. A fractured rib that has punctured the lung would most likely cause this.

➤ Equipment

You will need the following equipment:

Lead shields for other health-care workers
Lead shield(s) for patient
Standard Precautions equipment (gowns, gloves, face shields)
Various size cassettes
Expiration markers
Inspiration markers
Grids
Grid holder

➤ Recommendations

The first priority is to radiograph the patient's chest. This will be accomplished in the supine position. You will have to coordinate the exposure with the respiratory therapist to get full inspiration. It may be a good idea to ask the physician if an expiration chest radiograph would be warranted as well. If an expiration radiograph is requested, the expiration marker should be placed on the appropriate film holder. Once again, coordinate the exposure with the respiratory therapist.

The next radiograph could be either the lateral sternum or an oblique image of the sternum.

LATERAL STERNUM

Place a grid next to the patient's side. You may not have an option as to which lateral to take. This will be determined by the layout of the room and equipment. A grid holder should be used. Once again, coordinate the exposure with the respiratory therapist. The exposure should be taken on full inspiration.

MODIFIED OBLIQUE POSITION OF THE STERNUM

Place the patient supine and angle the central ray approximately 20 degrees mediolaterally toward the patient's left side. The central ray should be directed to the patient's sternum and exit in the midpoint of the grid. This projection should be part of your examination. Keep in mind, however, that because of your patient's injuries, it may be possible to x-ray the AP chest and lateral sternum only.

➤ Exposure Factors

- The patient should be accurately measured before determining the exposure factors. An exposure factor chart should be present in all examination rooms and control areas.
- The lateral sternum would require the use of a grid. Adjustments would have to be made according to the size of the patient's chest.

- The modified oblique sternum would also require the use of a grid. The exposure factors used for this would be determined by the presence of air or fluid.
- If a kVp greater than 90 is required to optimally penetrate the chest, a grid must be used.
- Optimal kVp ranges for this study:
  chest—120 kVp
  sternum—80 kVp

Case 3.2

➤ Goal

To successfully complete the procedure in a satisfactory manner.

➤ Observations

The patient is supine and keeps giggling. This could cause a problem with motion. The date of the patient's LMP has not been obtained. The physician wants all films taken supine.

➤ Equipment

You will need the following equipment:

Lead shields for other health-care workers
Lead shield(s) for the patient
Standard Precautions equipment (gowns, gloves, face shields)
Various size cassettes
Expiration markers
Inspiration markers
Grids
Grid holder

➤ Recommendations

First, obtain the date of the patient's LMP. Once you have determined and documented that she is not pregnant, develop an efficient order in which to take the films. They should be taken in the following order:

1. *Lateral cervical spine, horizontal central ray:* With a grid in the grid holder so that the long border of the grid is horizontal, have the patient inch her hands down on a sheet that has been placed around the bottom of her feet. This will help the shoulders to move down. Shield the patient's chest and pelvis with lead. Take the exposure on complete expiration. Have the film evaluated by the physician before continuing.
2. *Lateral thoracic spine, horizontal central ray:* With a grid in the grid holder, place the grid next to the patient's side. If the patient is able to lift up her arms so that her upper arms are perpendicular to the floor, her hands should be placed by her head. The exposure should be made on full inspiration. The grid should be placed lower than the back of the patient. This will allow the posterior part of the spine to be included on the film.
3. *Lateral lumbar spine, horizontal central ray:* With a grid in the grid holder, place the grid next to the patient's side. The exposure should be taken on expiration. The grid should be placed lower than the back of the patient. This will allow the posterior part of the spine to be included on the film.
4. *Coned spot lateral L5–S1, horizontal central ray:* Angle the central ray through the joint space using a caudal angle of approximately 8 degrees.

   The central ray is positioned over the patient. The following projections are taken:

AP cervical spine
AP open-mouth odontoid
AP thoracic spine
AP lumbar spine

5. *Modified oblique position cervical spine:* With the patient supine, place a grid cassette slightly under the patient's neck. Direct the central ray 45 degrees medially and 15 degrees cephalad. This should be directed to the level of C4. Repeat the same position for the opposite side.

➤ Exposure Factors

- The patient should be accurately measured before determining the exposure factors. An exposure factor chart should be present in all examination rooms and control areas.
- If the patient continues to giggle, this fact should be brought to the physician's attention, using established procedural protocols. The patient may be giggling simply over the silliness of her situation, but her inability to stop laughing could be indicative of brain injury. If motion becomes a problem, you should adjust your exposure factors for this. A large mA station should be used, along with a short exposure time.
- The following examinations will require the use of a grid:
  AP thoracic spine
  Lateral thoracic spine
  AP lumbar spine
  Lateral lumbar spine
  Oblique cervical spine
- The L5–S1 lumbar spot radiograph should be closely collimated, to reduce exposure to the patient and to enhance the visibility of detail.
- Optimal kVp ranges for this study:
  AP vertebral column—80 kVp
  lateral vertebral column—90 kVp

Case 3.3

➤ Goal

To successfully complete the procedure in a satisfactory manner.

➤ Observations

The patient is supine. There is a considerable amount of blood loss. Standard Precautions are required. His femur appears to be fractured, and his shoulder is out of alignment.

➤ Equipment

You will need the following equipment:

Standard Precautions equipment (gowns, gloves, goggles)
Cassettes of various sizes
Extremity cassettes
Several grids of various sizes
Grid holder
Radiolucent sponges, various sizes

➤ Recommendations

The first priority is to organize an efficient plan. Because of blood loss, the patient may be in danger of experiencing shock. The examination should proceed as follows:

1. *AP femur:* A large cassette is used. Make certain that both joints are included.
2. *AP thoracic spine:* Routine position.
3. *AP shoulder:* A large film should be used to include the entire clavicle, scapula, and upper arm.
4. *Lateral femur, horizontal central ray:* Place a large grid next to the patient's right femur. Make certain that the grid remains in the vertical position. Include from the knee joint up on this radiograph. The second radiograph should be of the hip. Use a grid as well for this position. Have the patient elevate his left leg. This can be accomplished by bending the knee and resting the foot on a sponge.
5. *Lateral thoracic spine:* A large grid is used. The patient will not be able to lift his right arm. Attempt to place the grid between the patient's chest and his arm. This will most likely require that a "swimmer's" lateral be included because you were not able to include the upper vertebrae on the lateral thoracic spine radiograph.
6. *Transthoracic lateral:* Place a grid next to the patient's right humerus. Have the patient elevate his left arm over his head. Direct the central ray horizontally across the patient's chest.
7. *AP projection of the hand:* Use one exposure per cassette. The central ray will be vertical for this radiograph. The cassette may be angled to accommodate the oblique position of the hand. The central ray should be perpendicular to the hand and, consequently, to the film. An oblique position of the hand may be attempted, using sponges if appropriate.
8. *Lateral radiograph of the hand:* The central ray should be placed in the horizontal position. This time, it will be directed from the opposite direction. The hand should be gently placed on a sponge with the edge of the sponge next to the patient's thumb. The cassette should be placed to extend below the border of the palmar surface of the hand.

➤ Exposure Factors

- The patient should be accurately measured before determining the exposure factors. An exposure factor chart should be present in all examination rooms and control areas.
- Keep in mind that this patient is very muscular and will require an increase in exposure factors. If the patient is in shock, there may be a concern regarding motion.
- Optimal kVp ranges for this study:
  femur, shoulder—70 kVp
  hand—50 to 60 kVp
  AP vertebral column—80 kVp
  lateral vertebral column—90 kVp

Case 3.4

➤ Goal

To complete the examination in an efficient manner.

➤ Observations

The woman is a psychiatric patient. She is sedated, and it does not appear that she can help hold the positions. There is a small amount of blood from her right elbow. Standard Precautions will be used.

➤ Equipment

You will need the following equipment:

Standard Precautions equipment (gowns, gloves, goggles)
Lead shields
Various size cassettes
Grid(s)
Grid holder
Tape

➤ Recommendations

The first priority is to formulate a plan for an efficient manner in which to examine the patient. You also need to know the date of the patient's LMP. Once you are certain that she is not pregnant, you will take the following radiographs:

1. *AP chest:* Attempt to awaken patient so that she can take in a deep breath.
2. *AP lumbar spine:* Use a large cassette to include the abdomen as well.
3. *AP right lower leg:* Include both joints.
4. *AP right elbow:* Gently turn her arm into the supine position. If she appears to be in pain, stop immediately.
5. *Axial projections of an os calcis:* The patient will not be able to hold the gauze. Instead, radiolucent sponges can be placed along the sides of the foot and sandbags propped up against the sponges.
6. *Lateral lumbar spine:* A grid that extends below the edge of the table will be needed.
7. *Lateral right lower leg:* The cassette can be placed along the medial aspect of the lower leg. Make certain that the posterior part of the leg is included on the cassette. It may be necessary to place the leg on a sponge.
8. *Lateral right elbow:* The elbow will probably not be flexed for this position. A horizontal central ray can be used. A sponge should be placed under the elbow. This will allow the elbow to be included on the cassette in its entirety. Attempt to have the humeral epicondyles perpendicular to the film. If this is not possible, take this radiograph so that it is 90 degrees from the AP radiograph.
9. *Lateral right os calcis:* Place an extremity cassette along the medial aspect of the patient's right os calcis. Place the os calcis on a sponge. Direct the central ray horizontally to the midpoint of the os calcis. It may be a good idea to include as much of the ankle and foot as possible.
10. *Lateral left os calcis:* Place the os calcis on a sponge. Place the cassette so that it is in contact with the medial aspect of the lateral os calcis. Direct the central ray horizontally to the midpoint of the os calcis.

➤ Exposure Factors

- The patient should be accurately measured before determining the exposure factors. An exposure factor chart should be present in all examination rooms and control areas.
- Keep in mind that you will be alternating between regular cassettes and extremity cassettes.
- Optimal kVp ranges for this study:
  femur, shoulder, lower leg—70 kVp
  elbow, os calcis—50 to 60 kVp
  AP vertebral column—80 kVp
  lateral vertebral column—90 kVp
  chest—120 kVp
  AP pelvis (abdomen)—80 kVp

Case 3.5

➤ Goal

To successfully complete the examination in a satisfactory manner.

➤ Observations

The patient is medicated but alert. He has burns across his scapulae. All radiographs should be made while he is recumbent. The physician states that the patient may turn slightly if he can tolerate it.

➤ Equipment

You will need the following equipment:

Standard Precautions equipment (gowns, gloves, goggles)
Lead shields
Radiolucent sponges
Grids
Grid holder

➤ Recommendations

The use of Standard Precautions is strongly recommended. Also, any dressing that has been placed on the burns may not be removed or contaminated in any way.

The chest radiograph should be made in the supine position even though the prone position would cause the patient the least amount of pain. Unfortunately, the prone position is not possible with this patient. The first priority is to organize the examinations. The following order is suggested:

1. *AP below diaphragm ribs:* The cassette is placed to include both rib areas. The exposure should be taken on complete expiration. This will allow the ribs below the diaphragm to be demonstrated.
2. *AP above diaphragm ribs:* The cassette is placed to include both rib areas. The exposure should be taken on complete inspiration. This will allow demonstration of all of the ribs above the diaphragm.
3. *AP right scapula:* The patient should be instructed as to the starting position of his arm. Gently, and with great patience, guide his arm so that the humerus is at a right angle to his thorax.
4. *Lateral right scapula:* With the patient's arm still over his head, instruct the patient to turn slightly to his left. Place a radiolucent sponge under the patient's slightly elevated right side (left posterior oblique [LPO] position). Gently palpate the patient's scapula, adjusting the degree of obliquity, until both borders of the scapula are superimposed.
5. *LPO ribs:* With the patient in the above position, instruct him to continue to roll onto his left side until he is in a 45-degree oblique position. The exposure should be taken on complete inspiration.
6. *Oblique sternum:* With the patient in the LPO position, x-ray the sternum.
7. *AP left scapula:* The patient is instructed to turn back into the supine position. Give gentle support during this process. Once he is in the supine position, again instruct him as to the position of his left arm. Gently, and with great patience, guide his arm so that the humerus is at a right angle to his thorax.
8. *Left lateral scapula:* With the patient's arm still over his head, instruct the patient to turn slightly to his right. Place a radiolucent sponge under the patient's slightly elevated left side (right posterior oblique [RPO] position). Gently palpate the patient's scapula, adjusting the degree of obliquity, until both borders of the scapula are superimposed.

9. *RPO ribs:* With the patient in the above position, instruct the patient to continue to roll onto his left side until he is in a 45-degree oblique position. The exposure should be taken on inspiration.
10. *Cross table lateral sternum:* Ask the patient to turn into the supine position. A grid is then placed in the grid holder and located between the patient's humerus and the lateral aspect of his thorax. The opposite arm can remain supine by the patient's side, provided that it will not obscure the sternal area. The central ray is directed horizontally and perpendicular to the patient's sternum.

Regarding positioning, have the patient move slowly and use radiolucent sponges. This will give the patient the support necessary to hold the positions. The LPO and RPO positions for the lateral scapulae have been suggested because these positions require less movement by the patient. In the routine that is suggested, the patient will turn the least possible number of times.

➤ Exposure Factors

- The patient should be accurately measured before determining the exposure factors. An exposure factor chart should be present in all examination rooms and control areas.
- The technique most likely will have to be increased because of the type and amount of physical work that this patient does. This is especially true of the shoulder and chest areas. For the chest and rib techniques, I would inquire if the patient is or was a heavy smoker. This could have an effect on the technique selected.
- Optimal kVp ranges for this study:
  scapulae, ribs, sternum—80 kVp

Case 3.6

➤ Goal

To successfully complete the examination as satisfactorily as possible.

➤ Observations

The patient must remain in the prone position for all radiographs. The physician will assist you in positioning the obliques.

➤ Equipment

You will need the following equipment:

Lead shields
Radiolucent sponges
Grids
Grid holder
Gowns (because of the horse manure)

➤ Recommendations

Because the physician has so clearly stated that the patient not be moved from the prone position, you have decided to perform the study in the following order, which is very efficient and much easier for the patient to tolerate. With this sequence of radiographs, the patient is placed in the oblique position one time only and the degree of obliquity is changed depending on what is to be demonstrated.

1. *PA projection, pelvis:* With the patient in the prone position, x-ray the pelvis. Make certain that the correct right or left marker has been used.

2. *PA projection of the lumbar spine:* Same as above.
3. *PA sacrum:* With the patient in the prone position, the central ray is angled 15 degrees caudally. (An AP projection requires a cephalic angle.)
4. *PA coccyx:* With the patient in the prone position, the central ray is angled 10 degrees cephalic. (An AP projection requires a caudal angle.)
5. *PA axial projection of the SI joints:* The central ray is directed 35 degrees caudally. (An AP axial projection requires a cephalic angle.)
6. *Lateral lumbar spine:* A grid is placed in a grid holder. This is placed along the lateral aspect of the patient's abdomen. The central ray is horizontal and is directed to the midpoint of the lumbar spine and the grid. The exposure is made on expiration to best demonstrate the upper lumbar vertebrae.
7. *Lateral sacrum and coccyx:* Attempt to demonstrate both structures on one radiograph. A grid is placed in a grid holder. It is placed alongside the patient and centered to the midpoint of the sacrum and coccyx. The central ray is horizontal and is directed to the midpoint of the sacral area. This would include the coccyx as well.

The following order is followed for the oblique radiographs:

1. *Right anterior oblique (RAO) lumbar spine:* Place an identifying left marker, marking the patient's left side (zypophyseal joints). The patient is obliqued 45 degrees.
2. *RAO SI joint:* Oblique the patient less than what was used on the lumbar spine (25 to 30 degrees). The central ray is directed perpendicular to the lower SI joint. This demonstrates the right SI joint.
3. *Left anterior oblique (LAO) lumbar spine:* Place an identifying right marker on the patient's right side (zypophyseal joints). The patient is obliqued 45 degrees.
4. *LAO SI joint:* Oblique the patient less than what was used on the lumbar spine (25 to 30 degrees). The central ray is directed perpendicular to the lowest SI joint. This demonstrates the left SI joint.

Note: *The zypophyseal joint demonstrated should be marked with the correct right or left marker; however, not all imaging departments do this. The important thing is that the radiographer knows which structure is being demonstrated. For example, in the instance when the patient is placed in the RAO position, the left zypophyseal joints are best demonstrated and the lowermost or right SI joint is demonstrated as well.*

➤ Exposure Factors

- The patient should be accurately measured before determining the exposure factors. An exposure factor chart should be present in all examination rooms and control areas.
- Lateral lumbar cross table: use a grid.
- Lateral sacrum and coccyx: use a grid.
- Oblique lumbosacral (LS) spine: use a grid.
- Optimal kVp ranges for this study:
  - *pelvis (abdomen), AP lumbar spine, lumbar obliques, AP sacrum, AP coccyx, SI joints (axial and obliques)—80 kVp*
  - *lateral vertebral column, lateral sacrum, lateral coccyx—90 kVp*

Case 3.7

➤ Goal

To complete the examination as satisfactorily as possible.

➤ Observations

The patient has numbness in his fingertips.

➤ Equipment

You will need the following equipment:

Cassettes
Various weights
Lead shields

➤ Recommendations

The patient is instructed to sit in a chair and not to move his head. It must be noted that the radiographer must handle this situation calmly to prevent undue anxiety to the patient. The physician is notified immediately regarding the patient's complaint of numbness in his fingertips. The physician will then determine what radiographs will be taken. The key to the successful completion on this radiographic examination is the physician's assessment of the patient. You have already used a proper assessment protocol in bringing the patient's fingertip numbness to the physician's attention. If the physician decides that there is the potential for possible spinal cord damage if the examination were to continue, he or she will call a stop to the procedure at this point. Your task will be complete.

The physician may decide to have you take a standing lateral cervical spine radiograph with no weights to more fully assess the patient. If the physician, after viewing the radiograph, decides that there is no discernible fracture or other trauma, the examination may continue. The examination is completed as follows:

1. *Lateral cervical spine:* With the patient in the erect position, direct the central ray perpendicular to the fourth cervical vertebra. Because of the patient's inability to hold weights, he can be instructed to exhale completely for the radiograph. This should help to depress the shoulders, thereby allowing visualization of the lower cervical vertebrae.
2. *Oblique cervical spine:* These radiographs can be taken with the patient in either a PA projection or an AP projection.
3. *AP cervical spine:* Because of the patient's injury, it may be a good idea to perform this examination in the erect position.
4. *Open-mouth odontoid projection:* This can also be taken in the erect position.

➤ Exposure Factors

- The patient should be accurately measured before determining the exposure factors. An exposure factor chart should be present in all examination rooms and control areas.
- Optimal kVp ranges for this study:
  vertebral column—80 kVp

Case 3.8

➤ Goal

To complete the examination in a satisfactory manner.

➤ Observations

The patient is elderly and supine. She is also asthenic and kyphotic. The patient's right hip and elbow are probably fractured. You anticipate that the patient will not be able to move either the right hip or the right elbow. Standard Precautions will be needed. The patient is alert and obviously nervous.

➤ Equipment

You will need the following equipment:

Standard Precautions equipment (gowns, gloves, goggles)
Extremity cassettes
Various size grids
Grid holder
Large block radiolucent sponge
Small radiolucent sponges
Lead shield

➤ Recommendations

The examination should be completed in the following order:

1. *AP pelvis:* You should begin this examination by taking an AP projection of the patient's pelvis. Her legs are not internally rotated because of your initial assessment of her physical condition. This should be noted for the radiologist.
2. *AP hip:* For this projection, use a larger cassette. This will demonstrate a fracture that could extend from the hip to the femoral area.
3. *AP elbow and AP forearm:* The first thing you need to do is assess the patient's ability to rotate and supinate her arm. You would then take an exposure of the patient's AP elbow, followed by the AP forearm (assuming that she can indeed rotate her arm). Use one cassette per position.
4. *Oblique elbow:* These radiographs would be obtained by placing the cassette under the patient's elbow and offsetting the cassette. For the lateral oblique, angle the central ray 45 degrees laterally. Direct the central ray to the midpoint of the cassette, allowing for the offset resulting from the central ray's angle. For the medial oblique, direct the central ray 40 degrees medially, providing that the patient can abduct her arm for the placement of the cassette.
5. *Lateral elbow and forearm:* Place a sponge under the patient's forearm and elbow. The edge of the sponge should be at the edge of the medial aspect of her arm. A cassette is placed along the medial aspect of the patient's elbow. The central ray is directed horizontally through the elbow. For the forearm, place the cassette along the medial aspect of the forearm and direct the central ray horizontally through the forearm in the same manner.
6. *Lateral hip:* First, make certain that the patient is covered with a sheet. Then, place a large grid cassette next to the lateral aspect of the patient's right hip. The cassette should be angled so that it is parallel with the femoral neck. The opposite leg should be lifted so that the unaffected femur can be placed perpendicular to the table top. This can be accomplished by using radiolucent sponges under the patient's foot.

➤ Exposure Factors

- The patient should be accurately measured before determining the exposure factors. An exposure factor chart should be present in all examination rooms and control areas.
- Keep in mind that the patient is elderly. She is also asthenic and kyphotic, which points to her being osteoporotic. Because of this, the kVp should be kept relatively low. The loss of bone mass or calcium content within the bones renders the bones easier to penetrate, and they are considered more radiolucent. It must be noted, however, that approximately 50 percent of the bone density must be lost before bone loss can be demonstrated on the radiographic image. With regard to the cross-table lateral hip, it will be difficult to demonstrate the right hip if the patient cannot be positioned so that her left femur is perpendicular. Increasing the kVp might be tempting, but the real correction would be to lift the patient's leg more. If this is not possible, then it is advisable to radiograph the patient using the axiolateral projection, Clements-Nakayama modification. This projection is used for patients that have bilateral hip injuries or a limitation of movement in the unaffected leg.

- Optimal kVp ranges for this study:
  elbow—50 to 60 kVp
  hip, pelvis—80 kVp

Case 3.9

➤ Goal
To successfully complete this examination in a satisfactory manner.

➤ Observations
The patient is a 51-year-old man. He is nonresponsive and has been involved in an automobile accident. He has abdominal injuries and possibly a head injury as well. The patient's abdomen appears to be very large. The patient has clear fluid coming out of his right ear.

➤ Equipment
You will need the following equipment:

Lead aprons and shielding for other health-care workers
Standard Precautions equipment (gloves, gown, face shield)
Grids
Grid holder
Various size cassettes
Tape

➤ Recommendations
Time is of greatest importance. It is recommended that you take the following radiographs in this order:

AP chest
Abdomen
Skull (Towne method)
AP skull
AP (Caldwell)
Lateral skull
Lumbar spine, lateral

Start with an AP projection of the patient's chest. This would be followed by the AP projection of the patient's abdomen. You might decide to take two radiographs, depending on the size of the patient's abdomen. For a large patient, it is recommended that radiographs be taken of the abdomen and that the cassettes be placed transverse across the patient's abdomen. The first radiograph would cover the upper portion of the abdomen, and the second would demonstrate the lower portion. The AP abdomen radiographs should demonstrate the lumbar spine as well. You should then take an AP axial (Towne method), which would demonstrate the base of the skull. Clear fluid coming from the ear can be the result of a fracture in the petrous area of the skull. This would be cerebrospinal fluid. You should then take an AP skull, and if the patient is stable enough, you might attempt an AP (Caldwell) projection. The remaining radiographs would be your lateral projections, and the central ray would be turned horizontally. A lateral skull and a lateral lumbar spine would be taken. The spine radiograph should be taken on a large film, and you would want to demonstrate as much of the abdomen as possible.

➤ Exposure Factors
- The patient should be accurately measured before determining the exposure factors. An exposure factor chart should be present in all examination rooms and control areas.

- If a patient has experienced trauma to the abdomen and the abdomen appears to be very large in relation to the patient's body, hemorrhage is a possibility. If this is the case, the abdomen will be very dense (much like abdominal ascites) and difficult to demonstrate. For the chest radiograph, you should keep in mind that the anesthesiologist will probably want to demonstrate the endotracheal tube for placement within the trachea. The skull examination will be pretty much routine, although the AP axial skull must demonstrate the base of the skull.
- Optimal kVp ranges for this study:
  chest—120 kVp
  abdomen—80 kVp
  skull—80 kVp

Case 3.10

➤ Goal

To successfully complete the procedure in a satisfactory manner.

➤ Observations

The patient is unresponsive and supine. The patient has multiple myeloma.

➤ Equipment

You will need the following equipment:

Lead shield (place on chest area and extend the shield to cover the pelvis)
Grid and grid holder
Tape
Radiolucent angle and block sponges
Standard Precautions equipment (gloves, gown, and face shield)

➤ Recommendations

Once all planning has been completed, place the patient in an AP position. Make certain that the patient's orbitomeatal line (OML) is perpendicular by placing a sponge under the patient's head if necessary. The following radiographs should then be completed:

1. *AP axial (Towne method)*
2. *AP skull*
3. *AP facial bones*
4. *AP mandible* (for mandibular rami)
5. *Acanthioparietal projection, reverse Water's method:* With the patient in the AP facial bones position, lift the patient's chin until the acanthiomeatal line is perpendicular. Direct the central ray perpendicular to the acanthion.
6. *Submentovertical projection for zygomatic arches:* Place a small block sponge under the patient's head. Place a grid in a vertical position at the vertex of the patient's head. The grid may be angled if necessary. Direct the central ray perpendicular to the infraorbitomeatal line (IOML) at a cephalic angle to the midpoint of the patient's head, at the level of the zygomatic arches. On completion of these radiographs, keep the small block sponge under the patient's head. Adjust the central ray to a horizontal position. Position the patient's head so that it remains in an AP skull position. The grid is placed in a grid holder. If the grid is not vertical, tape may be needed to hold it in the vertical position.

For the lateral projections, the central ray is turned to the horizontal position. A small radiolucent sponge is placed under the patient's head. A grid is placed in a grid holder; the cassette is placed next to the patient. The following projections are made:

1. *Lateral skull:* Direct the central ray to a point 2 in. above the external acoustic meatus.
2. *Lateral facial bones:* Direct the central ray to the uppermost zygoma.
3. *Axiolateral oblique projection for the ramus of the mandible:* Lift the patient's chin slightly. With her shoulders relaxed, place a cassette next to the patient's mandible. Direct the central ray 25 degrees cephalad. If the patient has large shoulders and is not able to relax them, position the patient so that the vertex of her head is angled toward the film. The central ray should be angled cephalad to separate the two sides of the mandible.

➤ Exposure Factors

- The patient should be accurately measured before determining the exposure factors. An exposure factor chart should be present in all examination rooms and control areas.
- Multiple myeloma is a malignant condition in which a tumor arises from the plasma cells of bone marrow. It is most often found in the flat bones of the skull, vertebrae, and pelvic bones. Spontaneous fractures can occur. This condition alters the bone mass by decreasing the atomic number of the tissue. This in turn requires a decrease in the technical factors used. It is important to note that approximately 50 percent of the bone loss must occur before a change will be demonstrated radiographically.
- In the AP axial (Towne method) make certain that the base of the skull, mandibular condyles, and zygomes are well demonstrated. Because of the density changes between the zygomas and the base of the skull, your technique will need to be adjusted accordingly.
- AP skull and facial bones are exposed in essentially the same position. The exposure factors should be adjusted to demonstrate these two distinct areas.
- AP mandible is basically the same position as above. The exposure factors should be adjusted to demonstrate the mandible.
- In the SMV the exposure factors used should demonstrate the zygomas, not the base of the skull.
- In the laterals the same position is essentially used in all instances. The exposure factors selected should be adjusted to demonstrate each distinct area.
- Optimal kVp ranges for this study:
  skull—80 kVp
  facial bones—<80 kVp

References

1. Drafke, MW: Trauma and Mobile Radiography. F. A. Davis, Philadelphia, 1990, pp 20–24.
2. Eisenberg, RL, and Dennis, CA: Comprehensive Radiographic Pathology. Mosby, St. Louis, 1995, pp 64–65.
3. Carlton, RR, and Adler, AM: Principles of Radiographic Imaging: An Art and a Science. Delmar, Albany, 1996, pp 264–278, 470.
4. Drafke, op cit, pp 90–100, 169–170.
5. Carlton and Adler, op cit, pp 236–246, 264–272, 470.
6. Ballinger, PW: Merrill's Atlas of Radiographic Positions and Radiologic Procedures, ed 8, Vols 1 and 2. Mosby, St. Louis, 1995, pp 350–351, 356–359, 364–371.
7. Carlton and Adler, op cit, pp 264–278, 343–356, 470.
8. Ballinger, op cit, Vol 1:pp 126–127, 129–131, 266–269, 352–353, 356–359.
9. Carlton and Adler, op cit, pp 264–273, 343–356, 470.
10. Ballinger, op cit, Vol 1:pp 101–103, 215–218, 234–237, 276–277, 367–369, 466–467.
11. Carlton and Adler, op cit, pp 247–252, 264–278, 470.
12. Ballinger, op cit, Vol 1:pp 164–165, 170–171, 408–409, 412–413, 426–429, 466–467.
13. Carlton and Adler, op cit, pp 264–278, 470.
14. Ballinger, op cit, Vol 1:pp 276–277, 364–366, 368–369, 378–379, 386–389.
15. Ibid, Vol 2:pp 327, 334–337, 342–343.
16. Carlton and Adler, op cit, pp 470.

17. Cullinan, AM, and Cullinan, JE: Producing Quality Radiographs, ed 2. Lippincott, Philadelphia, 1994, p 296.
18. Ballinger, op cit, Vol 1:pp 98–99, 100, 101–102, 104–105, 276–277, 286–287, 290–293.
19. Carlton and Adler, op cit, pp 250–263, 470.
20. Ballinger, op cit, Vol 1:pp 368, 466–467; Vol. 2, pp 38–39, 240–249.
21. Carlton and Adler, op cit, pp 256–258, 470.
22. Torres, LS: Basic Medical Techniques and Patient Care for Radiologic Technologists, ed 4. Lippincott, Philadelphia, 1993, p 121.
23. Ballinger, op cit, Vol 2:pp 246–250, 308–309, 342, 346–349.
24. Carlton and Adler, op cit, pp 265–266, 470.
25. Drafke, op cit, pp 142–146, 148.
26. Eisenberg and Dennis, op cit, pp 79–84.
27. Thomas, CL (ed): Taber's Cyclopedic Medical Dictionary, ed 18. F. A. Davis, Philadelphia, 1997, pp 1255, 1256.

Bibliography

Ballinger, PW: Merrill's Atlas of Radiographic Positions and Radiologic Procedures, ed 8, Vols 1–3.
Carlton, RR, and Adler, AM: Principles of Radiographic Imaging: An Art and a Science. Delmar, Albany, 1996
Cullinan, AM, and Cullinan, JE: Producing Quality Radiographs, ed 2. Lippincott, Philadelphia, 1994.
Drafke, MW: Trauma and Mobile Radiography. F. A. Davis, Philadelphia, 1990.
Eisenberg, RL, and Dennis, CA: Comprehensive Radiographic Pathology. Mosby, St. Louis, 1995.
Roberts, W, and Ross, B: Make It So: Leadership Lessons from Star Trek: The Next Generation. Pocket Books (Simon and Schuster), New York, 1995.
Thomas, CL (ed).: Taber's Cyclopedic Medical Dictionary, ed 18. F. A. Davis, Philadelphia, 1997.
Torres, LS: Basic Medical Techniques and Patient Care for Radiologic Technologists, ed 4,1993.

4

Critical Analysis of Radiographs

Now that you have completed the preceding sections of this book, you are ready to begin analyzing and critiquing the work that you have done. This section is designed to help you in that process by giving you an organized, systematic approach to follow. Performing these analyses on your films will help you to determine what, if anything, could have been changed to produce a better-quality radiograph. Additionally, it will help you to understand what you can change or correct and what is beyond your control.

Producing a quality radiograph requires that many different aspects of the examination be performed properly. For example, you may have perfectly positioned an abdomen radiograph, selected the proper film-screen combination, and set the proper technical factors, only to have the patient sneeze just as the exposure was made. Regardless of how well everything was done, the fact that there is a motion artifact on the finished radiograph renders the quality of that radiograph less than perfect (and perhaps, completely unacceptable for diagnostic purposes). Thus, a number of factors come into play when you are attempting to produce a quality radiograph. As a student, you must be able to recognize what these factors are, what affects them, and what you can do to control them in your favor.

The following section describes the major factors that affect the production of quality radiographs. It is not intended as an exhaustive discussion of these factors. There are many fine books on the market that provide far more detail on these factors. The following section should be regarded as a guide to be used when critiquing your radiographs.

RADIOGRAPHIC QUALITY

Radiographic quality is defined as the "exactness of representation of the anatomic structure on the radiograph within the useful density range."[1] Putting this more simply: Can you see the thing that you were aiming at, and does it look the way it is supposed to? A radiograph that exactly reproduces the anatomic part is called a *high-quality radiograph.* High quality is needed by radiologists to be able to make accurate diagnoses; therefore, nothing less than high radiographic quality should be your goal.[2] Let us now take a look at the various components that contribute to a high-quality radiograph.

Positioning

It should be evident that proper positioning of the anatomy that is being radiographed is vital to the production of a high-quality radiograph. In the critical analyses that follow, specific anatomic components pertaining to the radiographic examination in question are detailed. Failure to include these parts on the radiograph will automatically yield a poor-quality radiograph, regardless of how well you have managed to produce the other factors.

Exposure Factors

Optical Density

Optical density is defined as the blackening of the finished radiograph.[3] Its function is to provide something for the human eye to view. The differing optical densities present on a radiograph make up the image seen on that radiograph. This is primarily controlled by two other factors. Although source-image distance (SID) certainly affects the overall optical density of a radiograph (inverse square law), it is almost always a fixed distance. Thus, optical density is primarily controlled by the adjustment of milliampere seconds (mAs). This factor is directly controllable by you. The amount of mAs used for a given examination on a given patient depends on a number of items, including, but not limited to, the output of the radiographic unit, the film-screen speed, the intensifying screen type, processor time and temperature, generator phase, patient condition, and patient size. Aside from the patient factors, the other items are almost always standardized within a given imaging department or facility, thus reducing the number of factors over which you have direct control.

It should also be noted that optical density is also affected by the amount of peak kilovolts (kVp) used in the production of the finished radiograph. Kilovoltage is a primary influencing factor relating to density.

Radiographic Contrast

The function of contrast in the image is to make anatomic detail more visible.[4] It is defined as the variation in adjacent optical densities present on a radiograph and is the product of subject contrast (see below) and film contrast.[5] The primary controllable factor used to adjust the contrast scale is kVp. The correct scale of contrast often depends on the anatomic part being radiographed. For example, a standard plain abdomen radiograph would be of relatively high (short scale) contrast because of the low to moderate kVp range that would be used on an average patient. A high-density barium enema, performed on the same patient, would exhibit a low or long scale of contrast because of the relatively high kVp range that would be necessary to penetrate the barium-filled colonic structures. Additionally, patient size and tissue density can affect radiographic contrast. Because the contrast scale is what allows you to see the different anatomical structures, contrast is a major contributing factor in the production of a high-quality radiograph. It should also be noted that a given contrast scale that is deemed optimal for one radiograph may not be optimal for a different radiograph.

Image Detail

Image detail refers to the sharpness with which we see structures, particularly small ones, on the radiograph. This, in turn, can be broken down into two areas: sharpness of detail and visibility of detail. Sharpness refers to the amount of clarity of the image. This is completely controlled by geometric factors such as focal-spot size, SID, and object-image distance (OID), as well as film-screen combinations and motion. Visibility of detail refers to the ability to see the detail on the radiograph. Such things as fog can affect this. Thus, both sharpness and visibility of detail must be high to contribute to the overall radiographic quality.[6]

Distortion

Distortion is the misrepresentation of object size and shape on the finished radiograph. A distorted image is the result of misalignment between the radiographic tube and the part in question, the image receptor and the part in question, the radiographic tube and the receptor, or among all. Proper positioning and proper alignment are the major factors in reducing the degree of distortion present on a radiograph.[7]

Magnification

Although all structures on a radiograph are larger than the actual anatomic part that they represent, you should generally strive to keep the degree of magnification to the minimum level achievable. To do this, always keep the SID as large as possible and the OID as small as possible.[8]

Subject Contrast

Subject contrast is a factor over which you typically have little control (excluding examinations in which a compression band is used, for example), but it is a major component of the overall radiographic contrast that will be present on the finished radiograph. However, you need to consider various aspects of the patient's anatomy to be able to influence the finished radiographic contrast. Factors such as the part's thickness and the actual shape of the anatomic part in question also have a significant impact on the final radiographic contrast present. Knowledge of these factors and what to adjust in your exposure factors will significantly aid you in producing a high-quality radiograph.[9]

Sharpness

Any inadvertent movement of the patient, the x-ray tube, or the image receptor during exposure will result in motion on the finished radiograph. Always be sure to give clear, precise instructions to your patient and ensure that your equipment is properly secured before making the exposure. Above all, be sure to observe your patient to determine whether your instructions are being carried out.

Film Artifacts

An artifact is defined as any optical density on a radiograph that is not caused by the superimposition of anatomy in the primary radiograph beam.[10] Artifacts are thus undesirable on the finished radiograph. Artifacts can consist of virtually any common object. They can be grouped into three main categories: exposure artifacts, processing artifacts, and handling and storage artifacts.

EXPOSURE ARTIFACTS

Under this heading, you can list items such as earrings, necklaces, and eyeglasses that show up on a finished radiograph. This category also includes positioning errors, grid cutoff artifacts, double exposures, motion artifacts, and warped cassettes. This category is well within your ability to control. Always ensure that your equipment is working properly. Always pay attention to the alignment of the tube and grid. Be sure to check that your patient has removed all jewelry and eyeglasses before taking the exposure.[11]

PROCESSING ARTIFACTS

This type or artifact includes dirty rollers (which can produce sharp areas of increased or reduced optical density), chemical fog (which produces an overall graying or dulling of the image), roller marks (which includes guide shoe marks found on the leading or trailing edges of the film and Pi lines, occurring when there is dirt or a chemical stain on a roller), and wet-pressure sensitization (which produces small circular patterns of increased optical density).[12] Your imaging department has an ongoing quality-control program that monitors the performance of your film processors, thus reducing the chance of any of these artifacts occurring.

HANDLING AND STORAGE ARTIFACTS

Handling and storage artifacts include light or radiation fog, kink marks, static, and hyporetention.

LIGHT OR RADIATION FOG. A light leak in the darkroom, a faulty safelight, and films left in an examination room during a second exposure can all exhibit overall fogging. If you accidentally expose film to light or radiation, you should notify your supervisor immediately.

KINK MARKS. Improper handling or storage, either before or after exposure, causes kink marks. These marks appear to be made by pressing a fingernail into the film, but that is not the case. Kinking or bending the film causes it.

STATIC. Static artifacts most often occur during the winter months when humidity is low. Static appears as mark(s) resembling crowns, trees, or smudges. Using antistatic mats or humidifiers in the darkroom can reduce static.

HYPORETENTION. Finished radiographs can exhibit yellowing over time, caused by an inadequate wash cycle during processing. Again, a quality-control program would help to identify this type of problem.[13]

OBJECTIVES

On completing the preceding sections, the student will be able to evaluate a radiograph using the following criteria:

POSITIONING CRITIQUE
Superior aspect
Inferior aspect
Lateral aspects
Rotation

FILM IDENTIFICATION
Name/identifier
Date of examination
Appropriate markers

EXPOSURE FACTORS
Optical density
Contrast
Image detail
Distortion
Magnification
Sharpness
Film artifacts

DIRECTIONS FOR CRITICAL FILM ANALYSIS

The following sections describe radiographic examinations in several areas of the body. Each type of examination includes a Critical Film Analysis Form, which can be used to determine whether the radiograph in question can be considered high quality. Once you have examined the radiograph, fill out the accompanying form and compare your answers with those in this chapter.

Each examination or group of examinations in a body area is followed by a Clinical Challenge designed to promote further discussion and learning. You should attempt to answer these questions after completing the relevant examination(s). The answers to the Clinical Challenge questions are found at the end of this chapter (no peeking!).

CHEST

Posteroanterior

Requirements

The following must be included on all posteroanterior (PA) chest radiographs.

SUPERIOR ASPECT. The lower neck area and the entire lung apices must be included.

INFERIOR ASPECT. Both lower bases of the lungs, including the costophrenic angles of the lungs and ribs, must be included. Adequate inspiration is demonstrated by seeing 10 ribs.

LATERAL ASPECTS. The lungs must be seen in their entirety, apices to costophrenic angles.

ROTATION. Sternoclavicular joints are not rotated. If the patient has scoliosis, the spine will appear to be curved. The sternoclavicular joints will be rotated as well, as demonstrated by foreshortening and/or elongation of the clavicles. Adequate inspiration is demonstrated by seeing 10 ribs.

Exposure Critique

DENSITY. Density is acceptable if the thoracic vertebral bodies and intervertebral disk spaces are faintly visible through the shadow of the mediastinum. The images of the vertebral bodies and intervertebral disk spaces should not obscure the vascularity and pulmonary markings of the lungs.

CONTRAST. A low level of contrast is necessary to demonstrate the wide variety of anatomical densities present in the chest. A kVp level of 120 kVp (minimum) is recommended, along with the use of a high-ratio grid for adult patients.

IMAGE DETAIL. The level of detail is acceptable if fine details such as lung markings and peripheral pulmonary vasculature are demonstrated.

DISTORTION. If the anatomic structures are represented correctly on the radiograph, distortion can be said to be minimal. The sternoclavicular joints should be used to determine the presence of rotation or distortion. This would be determined by elongation or foreshortening of the clavicles.

MAGNIFICATION. Magnification should be minimal because of the large SID.

SHARPNESS. Because of the extremely short exposure times used, involuntary motion is not typically a problem. If motion is not present, pulmonary markings will appear distinct.

ARTIFACTS. The radiograph should be free of artifacts.

Film Identification

Some type of patient identifier, a date and time stamp, and appropriate markers (usually *R* and *L*) should be present on the radiograph. If the radiograph was done as a portable examination, it should be additionally marked as a portable. Also, the SID used, the *exact* time when the examination was performed, and the position that the patient was in should be noted on the radiograph.

Critical Film Analysis Form

EXAMINATION ☐

Positioning Critique

Specify the structures that must be included on the radiograph:

Superior Aspect	
Inferior Aspect	
Lateral Aspects	
How would rotation be demonstrated?	

Film Identification	Yes	No
Patient Name/Identifier Present?	☐	☐
Date/Time of Examination Present?	☐	☐
Appropriate Markers Present?	☐	☐

	Yes	No
Evidence of collimation?	☐	☐
Evidence of shielding?	☐	☐

Yes ☐ No ☐

Exposure Factors

		Yes	No
Density	Acceptable?	☐	☐
	Demonstrated by:		
Contrast	Acceptable?	☐	☐
	Demonstrated by:		
Recorded Detail	Acceptable?	☐	☐
	Demonstrated by:		
Distortion	Acceptable?	☐	☐
	Demonstrated by:		
Magnification	Acceptable?	☐	☐
	Demonstrated by:		
Motion Sharpness	Acceptable?	☐	☐
	Demonstrated by:		
Film Artifacts	Acceptable?	☐	☐
	Demonstrated by:		

Lateral

Requirements

The following must be included on all lateral chest radiographs.

SUPERIOR ASPECT. Apices must be included. Make certain that the patient's upper arms are not on the radiograph.

INFERIOR ASPECT. Bases of the lungs must be included. If the patient is placed in a perfect lateral position, the lung bases will be superimposed. However, it should be noted that the lung base farther away from the actual cassette/image receptor will exhibit increased magnification.

LATERAL ASPECTS. Anteriorly, a lateral image of the sternum is demonstrated and the ribs are superimposed, posterior to the vertebral column.

ROTATION. Bases of the lungs should be superimposed. It should be noted that some radiologists prefer slight rotation to demonstrate both lung bases free of superimposition.

Exposure Critique

DENSITY. Density is acceptable if the vascularity and pulmonary markings of the lungs are demonstrated.

CONTRAST. A low scale of contrast is necessary to demonstrate the wide variety of anatomical densities present in the chest. A kVp level of 120 kVp (minimum) is recommended, along with the use of a high-ratio grid for adult patients.

IMAGE DETAIL. The level of detail is acceptable if fine details such as lung markings and peripheral pulmonary vasculature are demonstrated.

DISTORTION. If the anatomic structures are represented correctly on the radiograph, distortion can be said to be minimal.

MAGNIFICATION. Magnification should be minimal because of the large SID.

SHARPNESS. Because of the extremely short exposure times used, involuntary motion is not typically a problem. If motion is not present, pulmonary markings will appear distinct.

ARTIFACTS. The radiograph should be free of artifacts.

Film Identification

Some type of patient identifier, a date and time stamp, and appropriate markers (usually *R* and *L*) should be present on the radiograph. Although it is a rare occurrence, if the radiograph was done as a portable examination, it should be additionally marked as a portable. Also, the SID used, the *exact* time when the examination was performed, and the position that the patient was in should be noted on the radiograph.

Note: *It is important to note that use of a grid is assumed. This demonstrates the lung markings, as well as pathological conditions such as pleural thickening. Few shades of gray will be seen if the kVp is too low. This will result in radiographic contrast that is too high and will produce a radiograph that will demonstrate the lungs but not the mediastinum. If you have selected a kVp that is too high, the lung markings will not be demonstrated because of the low-scale contrast that will be produced by the high kVp. In regard to pathology, if the patient has congestive heart failure (CHF), the exposure must be increased because of the increased amount of fluid present. If the patient has emphysema or chronic obstructive pulmonary disease, the exposure must be decreased because of the increased aeration of the chest.*

Critical Film Analysis Form

EXAMINATION ☐

Positioning Critique

Specify the structures that must be included on the radiograph:

Superior Aspect	
Inferior Aspect	
Lateral Aspects	
How would rotation be demonstrated?	

Film Identification	Yes	No
Patient Name/Identifier Present?	☐	☐
Date/Time of Examination Present?	☐	☐
Appropriate Markers Present?	☐	☐

	Yes	No
Evidence of collimation?	☐	☐
Evidence of shielding?	☐	☐

Yes ☐ No ☐

Exposure Factors

		Yes	No
Density	Acceptable?	☐	☐
	Demonstrated by:		
Contrast	Acceptable?	☐	☐
	Demonstrated by:		
Recorded Detail	Acceptable?	☐	☐
	Demonstrated by:		
Distortion	Acceptable?	☐	☐
	Demonstrated by:		
Magnification	Acceptable?	☐	☐
	Demonstrated by:		
Motion Sharpness	Acceptable?	☐	☐
	Demonstrated by:		
Film Artifacts	Acceptable?	☐	☐
	Demonstrated by:		

Clinical Challenge

1. What are two conditions that require both inspiration and expiration PA chest radiographs?

2. Why is it important to write the position of the patient and the time when the radiograph was taken on all portable chest radiographs?

3. On reviewing a chest radiograph, you notice that the patient's heart is located on his or her right side. What do you do?

4. For a portable chest radiograph on an infant, you notice that the cassette is very cold. In an effort to make the cassette warmer, you place a blanket on the cassette. Will this affect the radiographic quality of the radiograph?

5. During a portable chest examination you are unable to sit the patient in a true upright position. He appears to be at approximately a 45-degree angle. Should you direct the central ray perpendicular to the patient's chest and film?

See page 256 for answers.

ABDOMEN

Anteroposterior

Requirements

The following must be included on all anteroposterior (AP) abdomen radiographs.

SUPERIOR ASPECT. The liver shadow must be included.

INFERIOR ASPECT. The lower border of the pubic symphysis must be included. If the patient is a middle-aged man, the area approximately 1 inch below the pubic symphysis should be included to demonstrate the area of the prostate gland.

LATERAL ASPECTS. The radiograph must include the area to the lateral border of the ribs. The spine will be seen in the middle of the radiograph.

ROTATION. Rotation is not present if the spinous processes are seen in the middle of the vertebral bodies. The wings of the ilium will also appear to be symmetrical. Rotation of the patient's abdomen can be determined by the position of the spinous processes within the spine. The spinous process should be in the center. The ilium of the pelvis should be symmetrical.

Exposure Critique

DENSITY. Density is acceptable if the following soft tissue structures are visually demonstrated:

Lower border of the liver
Bilateral kidney shadows
Gas patterns in the bowels
Urinary bladder, if full
Psoas muscles

CONSTRAST. Contrast level should be wide enough to demonstrate the various bony and soft tissue structures within the abdomen. A mid to high kVp (70 to 80 kVp) range is recommended, depending on the film-screen combination used and the patient's size and pathology.

IMAGE DETAIL. The level of detail is acceptable if small structures such as kidney stones, bony trabeculae, or phleboliths are clearly demonstrated.

DISTORTION. If the anatomic structures are represented correctly on the radiograph, as demonstrated by the alignment of structures, distortion can be said to be minimal.

MAGNIFICATION. Magnification will increase with patient size.

SHARPNESS. No blurring is seen on the radiograph. An immobilization band, along with proper patient instruction to suspend respiration, could be used to reduce motion.

ARTIFACTS. The radiograph should be free of artifacts.

Film Identification

Some type of patient identifier, a date and time stamp, and appropriate markers (usually *R* and *L*) should be present on the radiograph.

Critical Film Analysis Form

EXAMINATION ☐

Positioning Critique

Specify the structures that must be included on the radiograph:

Superior Aspect	
Inferior Aspect	
Lateral Aspects	
How would rotation be demonstrated?	

Film Identification

	Yes	No
Patient Name/Identifier Present?	☐	☐
Date/Time of Examination Present?	☐	☐
Appropriate Markers Present?	☐	☐
Evidence of collimation?	☐	☐
Evidence of shielding?	☐	☐

Yes ☐ No ☐

Exposure Factors

		Yes	No
Density	Acceptable?	☐	☐
	Demonstrated by:		
Contrast	Acceptable?	☐	☐
	Demonstrated by:		
Recorded Detail	Acceptable?	☐	☐
	Demonstrated by:		
Distortion	Acceptable?	☐	☐
	Demonstrated by:		
Magnification	Acceptable?	☐	☐
	Demonstrated by:		
Motion Sharpness	Acceptable?	☐	☐
	Demonstrated by:		
Film Artifacts	Acceptable?	☐	☐
	Demonstrated by:		

Clinical Challenge

1. If a patient could not stand or sit for an erect abdomen radiograph, how would you modify your procedure?

2. Your patient has a history of alcoholism. You have been requested to take a radiograph of the patient's abdomen. You notice that the patient is jaundiced. While positioning the patient, you notice that his abdomen appears very distended, and you suspect ascites. How would you modify your technical factors to produce an acceptable radiograph?

3. Your patient is extremely obese. You are unable to palpate any of the common bony structures needed to correctly position the patient. What should you do?

4. On examination of a routine abdomen radiograph, you notice small microcalcifications in the right upper area of the patient's abdomen. What radiographs, if any, do you think the radiologist may request?

See page 256 for answers.

GI SERIES

Posteroanterior Stomach

Requirements

The following must be included on all PA stomach radiographs.

SUPERIOR ASPECT. The fundus of the stomach must be included and is commonly seen filled with air. The area of the distal esophagus should also be demonstrated.

INFERIOR ASPECT. The duodenum and the lower border of the stomach must be demonstrated.

LATERAL ASPECTS. The entire stomach must be demonstrated.

ROTATION. Rotation is not present if the spinous processes are seen in the middle of the vertebral bodies.

Exposure Critique

DENSITY. Density is acceptable if the overall optical density is greater than that of a nonbarium abdomen study.

CONTRAST. For single-contrast barium studies, a range of 100 to 120 kVp is recommended to penetrate the barium. For a double-contrast study (using air and thick barium), a range of 80 to 90 kVp is recommended. The above kVp ranges allow adequate barium penetration and visual demonstration of mucosal detail.

IMAGE DETAIL. The level of detail is acceptable if small structures such as rugae and bony trabeculae are clearly demonstrated.

DISTORTION. Distortion will be present because of the relatively free movement of the barium-filled stomach. However, this is an expected occurrence.

MAGNIFICATION. Magnification will increase with patient size.

SHARPNESS. No blurring is seen on the radiograph, as evidenced by the lack of motion artifact in the areas of the diaphragm and duodenal loop.

ARTIFACTS. The radiograph should be free of artifacts.

Film Identification

Some type of patient identifier, a date and time stamp, and appropriate markers (usually *R* and *L*) should be present on the radiograph.

Critical Film Analysis Form

EXAMINATION ☐

Positioning Critique

Specify the structures that must be included on the radiograph:

Superior Aspect	
Inferior Aspect	
Lateral Aspects	
How would rotation be demonstrated?	

Film Identification	Yes	No
Patient Name/Identifier Present?	☐	☐
Date/Time of Examination Present?	☐	☐
Appropriate Markers Present?	☐	☐

	Yes	No
Evidence of collimation?	☐	☐
Evidence of shielding?	☐	☐

Yes ☐ No ☐

Exposure Factors

		Yes	No
Density	Acceptable?	☐	☐
	Demonstrated by:		
Contrast	Acceptable?	☐	☐
	Demonstrated by:		
Recorded Detail	Acceptable?	☐	☐
	Demonstrated by:		
Distortion	Acceptable?	☐	☐
	Demonstrated by:		
Magnification	Acceptable?	☐	☐
	Demonstrated by:		
Motion Sharpness	Acceptable?	☐	☐
	Demonstrated by:		
Film Artifacts	Acceptable?	☐	☐
	Demonstrated by:		

Lateral Stomach

Requirements

The following must be included on all lateral stomach radiographs.

SUPERIOR ASPECT. The distal esophagus and air-filled fundus of the stomach must be included.

INFERIOR ASPECT. The lower border of the stomach must be included, along with the duodenum.

LATERAL ASPECTS. The pyloris, duodenum, and anterior portion of the stomach must be included, along with the posterior portion of the stomach.

ROTATION. Rotation will not be present if the vertebral bodies appear in a block shape and the posterior facets are superimposed.

Exposure Critique

DENSITY. Density is acceptable if the overall optical density is greater than that of a nonbarium abdomen study.

CONTRAST. For single-contrast barium studies, a range of 100 to 120 kVp is recommended to penetrate the barium. For a double-contrast study (using air and thick barium), a range of 80 to 90 kVp is recommended. The above kVp ranges allow adequate barium penetration and visual demonstration of mucosal detail.

IMAGE DETAIL. The level of detail is acceptable if small structures such as rugae and bony trabeculae are clearly demonstrated.

DISTORTION. Distortion will be present because of the relatively free movement of the barium-filled stomach. However, this is an expected occurrence.

MAGNIFICATION. Magnification will increase with patient size.

SHARPNESS. No blurring is seen on the radiograph, as evidenced by the lack of motion artifact in the areas of the diaphragm and duodenal loop.

ARTIFACTS. The radiograph should be free of artifacts.

Film Identification

Some type of patient identifier, a date and time stamp, and appropriate markers (usually *R* and *L*) should be present on the radiograph.

Critical Film Analysis Form

EXAMINATION ☐

Positioning Critique

Specify the structures that must be included on the radiograph:

Superior Aspect	
Inferior Aspect	
Lateral Aspects	
How would rotation be demonstrated?	

Film Identification	Yes	No
Patient Name/Identifier Present?	☐	☐
Date/Time of Examination Present?	☐	☐
Appropriate Markers Present?	☐	☐

	Yes	No
Evidence of collimation?	☐	☐
Evidence of shielding?	☐	☐

Yes ☐ No ☐

Exposure Factors

		Yes	No
Density	Acceptable?	☐	☐
	Demonstrated by:		
Contrast	Acceptable?	☐	☐
	Demonstrated by:		
Recorded Detail	Acceptable?	☐	☐
	Demonstrated by:		
Distortion	Acceptable?	☐	☐
	Demonstrated by:		
Magnification	Acceptable?	☐	☐
	Demonstrated by:		
Motion Sharpness	Acceptable?	☐	☐
	Demonstrated by:		
Film Artifacts	Acceptable?	☐	☐
	Demonstrated by:		

Right Anterior Oblique Stomach

Requirements

The following must be included on all right anterior oblique (RAO) stomach radiographs.

SUPERIOR ASPECT. The distal esophagus and fundus (filled with air) of the stomach must be included.

INFERIOR ASPECT. The entire inferior portion of the stomach must be included.

LATERAL ASPECTS. The pylorus and duodenum, including the proximal jejunum, must be included, along with the greater curvature of the stomach.

ROTATION. The duodenal bulb and pylorus are presented free of superimposition of the stomach.

Exposure Critique

DENSITY. Density is acceptable if the overall optical density is greater than that of a nonbarium abdomen study.

CONTRAST. For single-contrast barium studies, a range of 100 to 120 kVp is recommended to penetrate the barium. For a double-contrast study (using air and thick barium), a range of 80 to 90 kVp is recommended. The above kVp ranges allow adequate barium penetration and visual demonstration of mucosal detail.

IMAGE DETAIL. The level of detail is acceptable if small structures such as rugae and bony trabeculae are clearly demonstrated.

DISTORTION. Distortion will be present because of the relatively free movement of the barium-filled stomach. However, this is an expected occurrence.

MAGNIFICATION. Magnification will increase with patient size.

SHARPNESS. Under normal time settings, involuntary motion of the stomach should not be seen. However, this position increases the incidence of peristalsis, which may lead to motion artifacts. Motion would be evidenced by the presence of blurring in the areas of the diaphragm and duodenal loop.

ARTIFACTS. The radiograph should be free of artifacts.

Film Identification

Some type of patient identifier, a date and time stamp, and appropriate markers (usually *R* and *L*) should be present on the radiograph.

Note: *If the contrast medium selected is of the water-soluble type, the kVp range should be between 80 and 90 kVp. Remember that contrast media are used to increase the density of an organ. It is important to select the correct penetrability of the x-ray beam. This would require you to change the mAs accordingly.*

Critical Film Analysis Form

EXAMINATION ☐

Positioning Critique

Specify the structures that must be included on the radiograph:

Superior Aspect ☐

Inferior Aspect ☐

Lateral Aspects ☐

How would rotation be demonstrated? ☐

Film Identification	Yes	No
Patient Name/Identifier Present?	☐	☐
Date/Time of Examination Present?	☐	☐
Appropriate Markers Present?	☐	☐

	Yes	No
Evidence of collimation?	☐	☐
Evidence of shielding?	☐	☐

Yes ☐ No ☐

Exposure Factors

		Yes	No
Density	Acceptable?	☐	☐
	Demonstrated by:		
Contrast	Acceptable?	☐	☐
	Demonstrated by:		
Recorded Detail	Acceptable?	☐	☐
	Demonstrated by:		
Distortion	Acceptable?	☐	☐
	Demonstrated by:		
Magnification	Acceptable?	☐	☐
	Demonstrated by:		
Motion Sharpness	Acceptable?	☐	☐
	Demonstrated by:		
Film Artifacts	Acceptable?	☐	☐
	Demonstrated by:		

Clinical Challenge

1. Your patient's stomach is taking a long time to empty. In fact, the radiologist has left the room. What can you do to increase the activity of the patient's stomach?

2. What part of the stomach is not commonly seen in a PA projection on a patient with a hypersthenic body habitus?

3. In the following positions for stomach radiography, describe where the air and the contrast medium (barium) would be located: AP, PA, right lateral, RAO, and left posterior oblique (LPO).

See page 257 for answers.

BARIUM ENEMA

Anteroposterior

Requirements

The following must be included on all AP barium enema radiographs.

SUPERIOR ASPECT. The entire transverse colon, the hepatic flexure, and the splenic flexure must be included.

INFERIOR ASPECT. The entire rectum must be included.

LATERAL ASPECTS. The entire ascending and descending colon must be included.

ROTATION. Rotation is not present if the spinous processes are seen in the middle of the vertebral bodies. The wings of the ilium will also appear to be symmetrical. Rotation of the patient's abdomen can be determined by the position of the spinous processes within the spine. The spinous process should be in the center. The ilium of the pelvis should be symmetrical.

Exposure Critique

DENSITY. Density is acceptable if the overall optical density is greater than that of a nonbarium abdomen study. Structures such as the iliac crests should still be visible, whereas the renal borders and psoas shadows should not.

CONTRAST. For single-contrast barium studies, a range of 100 to 120 kVp is recommended to penetrate the barium. For a double-contrast study (using air and thick barium), a range of 80 to 90 kVp is recommended.

IMAGE DETAIL. The level of detail is acceptable if small structures such as mucosal folds, bony trabeculae, or diverticulum are clearly demonstrated.

DISTORTION. Distortion will be present because of the relatively free movement of the barium-filled bowel. However, structures such as the colonic flexures should appear to be symmetrical.

MAGNIFICATION. Magnification will increase with patient size.

SHARPNESS. There are two possible causes of motion on a barium enema study. The first is seen as an overall motion artifact caused by the patient's respiratory movements. Blurring of anatomical structures within the abdomen would show evidence of this. The second motion artifact is caused by spasms in the colon itself and would be demonstrated by blurring within the barium-filled colon.

ARTIFACTS. The radiograph should be free of artifacts.

Film Identification

Some type of patient identifier, a date and time stamp, and appropriate markers (usually *R* and *L*) should be present on the radiograph.

Critical Film Analysis Form

EXAMINATION ☐

Positioning Critique

Specify the structures that must be included on the radiograph:

Superior Aspect	
Inferior Aspect	
Lateral Aspects	
How would rotation be demonstrated?	

Film Identification	Yes	No
Patient Name/Identifier Present?	☐	☐
Date/Time of Examination Present?	☐	☐
Appropriate Markers Present?	☐	☐

	Yes	No
Evidence of collimation?	☐	☐
Evidence of shielding?	☐	☐

Yes ☐ No ☐

Exposure Factors

		Yes	No
Density	Acceptable?	☐	☐
	Demonstrated by:		
Contrast	Acceptable?	☐	☐
	Demonstrated by:		
Recorded Detail	Acceptable?	☐	☐
	Demonstrated by:		
Distortion	Acceptable?	☐	☐
	Demonstrated by:		
Magnification	Acceptable?	☐	☐
	Demonstrated by:		
Motion Sharpness	Acceptable?	☐	☐
	Demonstrated by:		
Film Artifacts	Acceptable?	☐	☐
	Demonstrated by:		

Lateral Rectum

Requirements

The following must be included on all lateral rectum radiographs.

SUPERIOR ASPECT. The entire rectum must be included, as well as the sigmoid area.

INFERIOR ASPECT. The distal rectum must be included.

LATERAL ASPECTS. The rectum must be included, along with the sigmoid colon.

ROTATION. Rotation can be determined by the position of the sacrum. The sacrum must be in profile, and the rectum should be seen anterior to the sacrum with no superimposition. Both hip joints should be superimposed. The hip joints would not be seen, however, if a gonadal shield is used properly.

Exposure Critique

DENSITY. Density is acceptable if the overall optical density is greater than that of a nonbarium abdomen study. Structures such as the iliac crests should still be visible, whereas the renal borders and psoas shadows should not.

CONTRAST. For single-contrast barium studies, a range of 100 to 120 kVp is recommended to penetrate the barium. For a double-contrast study (using air and thick barium), a range of 80 to 90 kVp is recommended.

IMAGE DETAIL. The level of detail is acceptable if small structures such as mucosal folds, bony trabeculae, or diverticulum are clearly demonstrated.

DISTORTION. Distortion will be present because of the relatively free movement of the barium-filled bowel. However, structures such as the colonic flexures should appear to be symmetrical.

MAGNIFICATION. Magnification will increase with patient size.

SHARPNESS. There are two possible causes of motion on a barium enema study. The first is seen as an overall motion artifact caused by the patient's respiratory movements. Blurring of anatomical structures within the abdomen would show evidence of this. The second motion artifact is caused by spasms in the colon itself and would be demonstrated by blurring within the barium-filled colon.

ARTIFACTS. The radiograph should be free of artifacts.

Film Identification

Some type of patient identifier, a date and time stamp, and appropriate markers (usually *R* and *L*) should be present on the radiograph.

Critical Film Analysis Form

EXAMINATION ☐

Positioning Critique

Specify the structures that must be included on the radiograph:

Superior Aspect	
Inferior Aspect	
Lateral Aspects	
How would rotation be demonstrated?	

Film Identification

	Yes	No
Patient Name/Identifier Present?	☐	☐
Date/Time of Examination Present?	☐	☐
Appropriate Markers Present?	☐	☐
Evidence of collimation?	☐	☐
Evidence of shielding?	☐	☐

Yes ☐ No ☐

Exposure Factors

		Yes	No
Density	Acceptable?	☐	☐
	Demonstrated by:		
Contrast	Acceptable?	☐	☐
	Demonstrated by:		
Recorded Detail	Acceptable?	☐	☐
	Demonstrated by:		
Distortion	Acceptable?	☐	☐
	Demonstrated by:		
Magnification	Acceptable?	☐	☐
	Demonstrated by:		
Motion Sharpness	Acceptable?	☐	☐
	Demonstrated by:		
Film Artifacts	Acceptable?	☐	☐
	Demonstrated by:		

Posteroanterior Axial Projection of Colon

Requirements

The following must be included on all posteroanterior axial projections of the colon.

SUPERIOR ASPECT. Attempt to include as much of the colon as possible. It is not necessary to include the transverse flexures on this projection.

INFERIOR ASPECT. The entire rectosigmoid portion must be included. Ideally, the enema tip has been removed.

LATERAL ASPECTS. The entire rectosigmoid portion must be included. Attempt to include as much of the ascending and descending colon as possible.

ROTATION. Rotation is minimal if the rectosigmoid portion is seen in the middle of the radiograph.

Exposure Critique

DENSITY. Density is acceptable if the overall optical density is greater than that of a nonbarium abdomen study. Structures such as the iliac crests should still be visible, whereas the renal borders and psoas shadows should not.

CONTRAST. For single-contrast barium studies, a range of 100 to 120 kVp is recommended to penetrate the barium. For a double-contrast study (using air and thick barium), a range of 80 to 90 kVp is recommended.

IMAGE DETAIL. The level of detail is acceptable if small structures such as mucosal folds, bony trabeculae, or diverticulum are clearly demonstrated.

DISTORTION. Because of the angulation of the central ray, distortion is deliberately used to elongate the rectosigmoid colon.

MAGNIFICATION. Magnification will increase with patient size.

SHARPNESS. There are two possible causes of motion in a barium enema study. The first is seen as an overall motion artifact caused by the patient's respiratory movements. Blurring of anatomical structures within the abdomen would show evidence of this. The second motion artifact is caused by spasms in the colon itself and would be demonstrated by blurring within the barium-filled colon.

ARTIFACTS. The radiograph should be free of any artifacts.

Film Identification

Some type of patient identifier, a date and time stamp, and appropriate markers (usually *R* and *L*) should be present on the radiograph.

Critical Film Analysis Form

EXAMINATION ☐

Positioning Critique

Specify the structures that must be included on the radiograph:

Superior Aspect ☐

Inferior Aspect ☐

Lateral Aspects ☐

How would rotation be demonstrated? ☐

Film Identification

	Yes	No
Patient Name/Identifier Present?	☐	☐
Date/Time of Examination Present?	☐	☐
Appropriate Markers Present?	☐	☐
Evidence of collimation?	☐	☐
Evidence of shielding?	☐	☐

Yes ☐ No ☐

Exposure Factors

		Yes	No
Density	Acceptable?	☐	☐
	Demonstrated by:		
Contrast	Acceptable?	☐	☐
	Demonstrated by:		
Recorded Detail	Acceptable?	☐	☐
	Demonstrated by:		
Distortion	Acceptable?	☐	☐
	Demonstrated by:		
Magnification	Acceptable?	☐	☐
	Demonstrated by:		
Motion Sharpness	Acceptable?	☐	☐
	Demonstrated by:		
Film Artifacts	Acceptable?	☐	☐
	Demonstrated by:		

Clinical Challenge

1. If the patient is not able to turn prone for a PA axial projection, what projection can be used instead?

2. Name two projections that demonstrate both the anterior and posterior walls of the rectum.

3. Name a common positioning error found on AP projections of the colon for a patient who has a hyposthenic body habitus.

4. Why is a high kVp exposure used for a regular barium examination?

See page 257 for answers.

CERVICAL SPINE

Lateral

Requirements

The following must be included on all lateral cervical spine radiographs.

SUPERIOR ASPECT. The first cervical vertebra must be included.

INFERIOR ASPECT. The seventh cervical vertebra must be included. In patients who have eight vertebrae, all eight must be included.

LATERAL ASPECTS. The entire cervical spine must be included. Make certain that the angle of the mandible does not overlap the anterior aspect of C2 and C3. This can be corrected by lifting the patient's chin.

ROTATION. Rotation is present when the spinous processes are not in profile.

Exposure Critique

DENSITY. Density is acceptable if the bony and soft tissue structures (sternocleidomastoid muscles) in the cervical region are visually demonstrated.

CONTRAST. The contrast scale should be wide enough to demonstrate the detail of the bony vertebrae and soft tissue musculature within the neck.

IMAGE DETAIL. The level of detail is acceptable if small structures such as articular facets and intervertebral disk spaces are clearly demonstrated.

DISTORTION. Distortion will be present if there is abnormal foreshortening or elongation of vertebral structures such as the spinous processes.

MAGNIFICATION. Magnification should be minimized by the use of an increased SID (typically, 72 inches) to offset the inherent increase in the OID caused by the patient's shoulder being in contact with the image receptor.

SHARPNESS. Motion will be evident if blurring is seen in the vertebral trabeculae.

ARTIFACTS. The radiograph should be free of artifacts.

Film Identification

Some type of patient identifier, a date and time stamp, and appropriate markers (usually *R* and *L*) should be present on the radiograph.

Critical Film Analysis Form

EXAMINATION [ ]

Positioning Critique

Specify the structures that must be included on the radiograph:

Superior Aspect	
Inferior Aspect	
Lateral Aspects	
How would rotation be demonstrated?	

Film Identification	Yes	No
Patient Name/Identifier Present?	☐	☐
Date/Time of Examination Present?	☐	☐
Appropriate Markers Present?	☐	☐

	Yes	No
Evidence of collimation?	☐	☐
Evidence of shielding?	☐	☐

Yes ☐ No ☐

Exposure Factors

		Yes	No
Density	Acceptable?	☐	☐
	Demonstrated by:		
Contrast	Acceptable?	☐	☐
	Demonstrated by:		
Recorded Detail	Acceptable?	☐	☐
	Demonstrated by:		
Distortion	Acceptable?	☐	☐
	Demonstrated by:		
Magnification	Acceptable?	☐	☐
	Demonstrated by:		
Motion Sharpness	Acceptable?	☐	☐
	Demonstrated by:		
Film Artifacts	Acceptable?	☐	☐
	Demonstrated by:		

Anteroposterior

Requirements

The following must be included on all AP cervical spine radiographs.

SUPERIOR ASPECT. The third cervical vertebra must be included.

INFERIOR ASPECT. The second thoracic vertebra must be included.

LATERAL ASPECTS. The entire cervical spine must be included, along with the medial portion of the first and second ribs.

ROTATION. Rotation will be demonstrated if the spinous processes are not centered in the middle of the vertebral body.

Note: *If the patient's head is hyperextended, the occipital bone will be projected into the upper spine area. If the patient's head is not extended, the mandible will be projected into the spine. To prevent superimposition as described above, the patient's chin is lifted until a perpendicular line can be drawn connecting the occlusal plane of the upper teeth and the mastoid tips.*

Exposure Critique

DENSITY. Density is acceptable if the bony and soft tissue structures (sternocleidomastoid muscles) in the cervical region are visually demonstrated.

CONTRAST. The contrast scale should be wide enough to demonstrate the detail of the bony vertebrae and soft tissue musculature within the neck.

IMAGE DETAIL. The level of detail is acceptable if small structures such as the interpediculate spaces and intervertebral disk spaces are clearly demonstrated.

DISTORTION. Distortion will be present if there is abnormal foreshortening or elongation of vertebral structures such as the transverse processes.

MAGNIFICATION. Magnification will increase with patient size because of the increased OID.

SHARPNESS. Motion will be evident if blurring is seen in the vertebral trabeculae.

ARTIFACTS. The radiograph should be free of artifacts.

Film Identification

Some type of patient identifier, a date and time stamp, and appropriate markers (usually *R* and *L*) should be present on the radiograph.

Critical Film Analysis Form

EXAMINATION ☐

Positioning Critique

Specify the structures that must be included on the radiograph:

Superior Aspect	
Inferior Aspect	
Lateral Aspects	
How would rotation be demonstrated?	

Film Identification	Yes	No
Patient Name/Identifier Present?	☐	☐
Date/Time of Examination Present?	☐	☐
Appropriate Markers Present?	☐	☐

	Yes	No
Evidence of collimation?	☐	☐
Evidence of shielding?	☐	☐

Yes ☐ No ☐

Exposure Factors

		Yes	No
Density	Acceptable?	☐	☐
	Demonstrated by:		
Contrast	Acceptable?	☐	☐
	Demonstrated by:		
Recorded Detail	Acceptable?	☐	☐
	Demonstrated by:		
Distortion	Acceptable?	☐	☐
	Demonstrated by:		
Magnification	Acceptable?	☐	☐
	Demonstrated by:		
Motion Sharpness	Acceptable?	☐	☐
	Demonstrated by:		
Film Artifacts	Acceptable?	☐	☐
	Demonstrated by:		

Oblique

Requirements

The following must be included on all oblique cervical spine radiographs.

SUPERIOR ASPECT. The C1 vertebra must be included.

INFERIOR ASPECT. The T1 vertebra must be included.

LATERAL ASPECTS. All aspects of the spine must be included.

ROTATION. The spine is obliqued correctly when the intervertebral spaces are open and the spine is not obscured by the angle of the mandible when the chin is lifted.

Exposure Critique

DENSITY. Density is acceptable if the bony and soft tissue structures (sternocleidomastoid muscles) in the cervical region are visually demonstrated.

CONTRAST. The contrast scale should be wide enough to demonstrate the detail of the bony vertebrae and soft tissue musculature within the neck.

IMAGE DETAIL. The level of detail is acceptable if small structures such as intervertebral foramina and pedicles are clearly demonstrated.

DISTORTION. Distortion of vertebral structures such as the transverse processes will be present on a correctly positioned oblique. However, this is acceptable in this projection.

MAGNIFICATION. Magnification will increase with patient size because of the increased OID.

SHARPNESS. Motion will be evident if blurring is seen in the vertebral trabeculae.

ARTIFACTS. The radiograph should be free of artifacts.

Film Identification

Some type of patient identifier, a date and time stamp, and appropriate markers (usually *R* and *L*) should be present on the radiograph.

Critical Film Analysis Form

EXAMINATION ☐

Positioning Critique

Specify the structures that must be included on the radiograph:

Superior Aspect	
Inferior Aspect	
Lateral Aspects	
How would rotation be demonstrated?	

Film Identification

	Yes	No
Patient Name/Identifier Present?	☐	☐
Date/Time of Examination Present?	☐	☐
Appropriate Markers Present?	☐	☐

	Yes	No
Evidence of collimation?	☐	☐
Evidence of shielding?	☐	☐

Yes ☐ No ☐

Exposure Factors

		Yes	No
Density	Acceptable?	☐	☐
	Demonstrated by:		
Contrast	Acceptable?	☐	☐
	Demonstrated by:		
Recorded Detail	Acceptable?	☐	☐
	Demonstrated by:		
Distortion	Acceptable?	☐	☐
	Demonstrated by:		
Magnification	Acceptable?	☐	☐
	Demonstrated by:		
Motion Sharpness	Acceptable?	☐	☐
	Demonstrated by:		
Film Artifacts	Acceptable?	☐	☐
	Demonstrated by:		

Anteroposterior Open-Mouth C1 and C2

Requirements

The following must be included on all open-mouth C1 and C2 radiographs.

SUPERIOR ASPECT. The entire odontoid process is demonstrated free of superimposition. The teeth do not obscure the odontoid process. This can be determined before making the exposure by drawing a line from the upper edge of the incisors to the occipital bone and ensuring that this line is perpendicular to the image receptor.

INFERIOR ASPECT. The joint spaces of C1 and C2 are open.

LATERAL ASPECTS. The entire odontoid process is demonstrated free of superimposition.

ROTATION. C1–2 joint spaces will not be symmetrical if the spine is rotated.

Exposure Critique

DENSITY. Density is acceptable if the bony and soft tissue structures (sternocleidomastoid muscles) in the cervical region are visually demonstrated.

CONTRAST. The contrast scale should be wide enough to demonstrate the detail of the bony vertebrae and soft tissue musculature within the neck.

IMAGE DETAIL. The level of detail is acceptable if small structures such as the articulation between C1 and C2 and the dens are clearly demonstrated.

DISTORTION. Distortion is present if there is abnormal elongation or foreshortening of the odontoid process.

MAGNIFICATION. Magnification should be minimal in all cases because of minimal OID.

SHARPNESS. Motion will be evident if blurring is seen in the vertebral trabeculae.

ARTIFACTS. The radiograph should be free of artifacts.

Notes: *Never remove a patient's cervical collar or move a patient who has sustained neck trauma until permission to do so has been given by the physician. If performing a cervical spine on a young female patient, shield her breasts as well as her gonads. For horizontal central ray projections (cross-table), obtain permission from the physician before applying traction to the patient's arms.*

Critical Film Analysis Form

EXAMINATION ☐

Positioning Critique

Specify the structures that must be included on the radiograph:

Superior Aspect	
Inferior Aspect	
Lateral Aspects	
How would rotation be demonstrated?	

Film Identification	Yes	No
Patient Name/Identifier Present?	☐	☐
Date/Time of Examination Present?	☐	☐
Appropriate Markers Present?	☐	☐

	Yes	No
Evidence of collimation?	☐	☐
Evidence of shielding?	☐	☐

Yes ☐ No ☐

Exposure Factors

		Yes	No
Density	Acceptable?	☐	☐
	Demonstrated by:		
Contrast	Acceptable?	☐	☐
	Demonstrated by:		
Recorded Detail	Acceptable?	☐	☐
	Demonstrated by:		
Distortion	Acceptable?	☐	☐
	Demonstrated by:		
Magnification	Acceptable?	☐	☐
	Demonstrated by:		
Motion Sharpness	Acceptable?	☐	☐
	Demonstrated by:		
Film Artifacts	Acceptable?	☐	☐
	Demonstrated by:		

Clinical Challenge

1. When an automatic exposure control (AEC) device is used during radiography of the cervical spine, what common positioning mistake is often made?

2. A clay shoveler's fracture is an injury of the type received by workers who shovel heavy clay.[14] What part of the cervical spine is involved in this fracture?

3. What projection demonstrates the presence of cervical ribs?

4. You have been instructed to demonstrate the posterior elements of the cervical spine. What radiographs will you take?

See page 257 for answers.

LUMBOSACRAL SPINE

Anteroposterior

Requirements

The following must be included on all AP lumbosacral spine radiographs.

SUPERIOR ASPECT. The T12 vertebra must be included in its entirety.

INFERIOR ASPECT. The sacroiliac joints must be included in their entirety.

LATERAL ASPECTS. The entire lumbar spine is placed in the middle of the radiograph. Kidney shadows must be included.

ROTATION. Rotation is present when the spinous processes are not located within the middle of the vertebrae.

Exposure Critique

DENSITY. Density is acceptable if the bony trabeculae and soft tissue structures such as the psoas shadows in the lumbosacral region are visually demonstrated.

CONTRAST. Contrast scale should be low enough to demonstrate the bony trabeculae and soft tissue structures such as the psoas shadows in the lumbosacral region. A kVp range of 70 to 80 kVp is recommended.

IMAGE DETAIL. The level of detail is acceptable if small structures such as transverse processes, psoas muscles, and intervertebral disk spaces are clearly demonstrated.

DISTORTION. If the anatomic structures are represented correctly on the radiograph, distortion can be said to be minimal. Because of the natural lordosis of the lumbosacral spine, it is strongly recommended that the patient be positioned with the knees flexed.

MAGNIFICATION. Magnification will increase with increasing patient size.

SHARPNESS. Motion is present if structures such as the bony trabeculae appear blurred.

ARTIFACTS. The radiograph should be free of artifacts.

Film Identification

Some type of patient identifier, a date and time stamp, and appropriate markers (usually *R* and *L*) should be present on the radiograph.

Critical Film Analysis Form

EXAMINATION ☐

Positioning Critique

Specify the structures that must be included on the radiograph:

Superior Aspect	
Inferior Aspect	
Lateral Aspects	
How would rotation be demonstrated?	

Film Identification	Yes	No
Patient Name/Identifier Present?	☐	☐
Date/Time of Examination Present?	☐	☐
Appropriate Markers Present?	☐	☐

	Yes	No
Evidence of collimation?	☐	☐
Evidence of shielding?	☐	☐

Yes ☐ No ☐

Exposure Factors

		Yes	No
Density	Acceptable?	☐	☐
	Demonstrated by:		
Contrast	Acceptable?	☐	☐
	Demonstrated by:		
Recorded Detail	Acceptable?	☐	☐
	Demonstrated by:		
Distortion	Acceptable?	☐	☐
	Demonstrated by:		
Magnification	Acceptable?	☐	☐
	Demonstrated by:		
Motion Sharpness	Acceptable?	☐	☐
	Demonstrated by:		
Film Artifacts	Acceptable?	☐	☐
	Demonstrated by:		

Lateral

Requirements

The following must be included on all lateral lumbosacral radiographs:

SUPERIOR ASPECT. The entire T12 vertebra must be included.

INFERIOR ASPECT. As much of the sacrum as possible must be included.

LATERAL ASPECTS. The entire lumbar spine is placed in the middle of the radiograph. Kidney shadows must be included.

ROTATION. Posterior or anterior rotation: spinous processes not seen in profile and intervertebral foramina will not appear open.

Superior or inferior rotation of the spine: the vertebral bodies will not be seen as sharp, squared-off images.

Exposure Critique

DENSITY. Density is acceptable if the bony trabeculae and soft tissue structures such as the abdominal musculature in the lumbosacral region are visually demonstrated.

CONTRAST. Contrast scale should be low enough to demonstrate the bony trabeculae and soft tissue structures such as the abdominal musculature in the lumbosacral region. A kVp range of 70 to 80 kVp is recommended.

IMAGE DETAIL. The level of detail is acceptable if small structures such as the intervertebral foramina L1–4 are clearly demonstrated in profile.

DISTORTION. Distortion is present if there is demonstrated abnormal elongation or foreshortening of anatomical structures such as the vertebral bodies.

MAGNIFICATION. Magnification will increase with increasing patient size because of increased OID.

SHARPNESS. Motion is present if structures such as the bony trabeculae appear blurred.

ARTIFACTS. The radiograph should be free of artifacts.

Film Identification

Some type of patient identifier, a date and time stamp, and appropriate markers (usually *R* and *L*) should be present on the radiograph.

Critical Film Analysis Form

EXAMINATION ☐

Positioning Critique

Specify the structures that must be included on the radiograph:

Superior Aspect	
Inferior Aspect	
Lateral Aspects	
How would rotation be demonstrated?	

Film Identification

	Yes	No
Patient Name/Identifier Present?	☐	☐
Date/Time of Examination Present?	☐	☐
Appropriate Markers Present?	☐	☐

	Yes	No
Evidence of collimation?	☐	☐
Evidence of shielding?	☐	☐

Yes ☐ No ☐

Exposure Factors

		Yes	No
Density	Acceptable?	☐	☐
	Demonstrated by:		
Contrast	Acceptable?	☐	☐
	Demonstrated by:		
Recorded Detail	Acceptable?	☐	☐
	Demonstrated by:		
Distortion	Acceptable?	☐	☐
	Demonstrated by:		
Magnification	Acceptable?	☐	☐
	Demonstrated by:		
Motion Sharpness	Acceptable?	☐	☐
	Demonstrated by:		
Film Artifacts	Acceptable?	☐	☐
	Demonstrated by:		

L5–S1 Lumbosacral Junction

Requirements

The following must be included on all L5–S1 lumbosacral junction radiographs.

SUPERIOR ASPECT. The entire L5 vertebra must be demonstrated.

INFERIOR ASPECT. The upper half of the sacrum must be included.

LATERAL ASPECTS. The anterior sacrum and the anterior body of L5 must be included. Posteriorly, the spinous process of L5 must be included, along with the posterior aspect of the sacrum.

ROTATION. Anterior to posterior rotation is seen when the spinous process of L5 is not in profile. Superior to inferior rotation is seen when the joint space is not clearly opened.

Exposure Critique

DENSITY. Density is acceptable if the bony trabeculae and soft tissue structures such as the abdominal musculature in the lumbosacral region are visually demonstrated.

CONTRAST. Contrast scale should be low enough to demonstrate the bony trabeculae and soft tissue structures such as the abdominal musculature in the lumbosacral region. A kVp range of 70 to 80 kVp is recommended.

IMAGE DETAIL. The level of detail is acceptable if the lowermost border of L5 and the upper border of the sacrum are seen as clearly defined edges.

DISTORTION. Distortion can be said to be minimal if the L5–S1 joint space is open.

MAGNIFICATION. Magnification will increase with increasing patient size because of increasing OID.

SHARPNESS. Motion is present if structures such as the bony trabeculae appear blurred.

ARTIFACTS. The radiograph should be free of artifacts.

Film Identification

Some type of patient identifier, a date and time stamp, and appropriate markers (usually *R* and *L*) should be present on the radiograph.

Note: *Lumbosacral spine radiographs should be taken on expiration.*

Critical Film Analysis Form

EXAMINATION ☐

Positioning Critique

Specify the structures that must be included on the radiograph:

Superior Aspect	
Inferior Aspect	
Lateral Aspects	
How would rotation be demonstrated?	

Film Identification

	Yes	No
Patient Name/Identifier Present?	☐	☐
Date/Time of Examination Present?	☐	☐
Appropriate Markers Present?	☐	☐

	Yes	No
Evidence of collimation?	☐	☐
Evidence of shielding?	☐	☐

Yes ☐ No ☐

Exposure Factors

		Yes	No
Density	Acceptable?	☐	☐
	Demonstrated by:		
Contrast	Acceptable?	☐	☐
	Demonstrated by:		
Recorded Detail	Acceptable?	☐	☐
	Demonstrated by:		
Distortion	Acceptable?	☐	☐
	Demonstrated by:		
Magnification	Acceptable?	☐	☐
	Demonstrated by:		
Motion Sharpness	Acceptable?	☐	☐
	Demonstrated by:		
Film Artifacts	Acceptable?	☐	☐
	Demonstrated by:		

Clinical Challenge

1. Your patient is a large elderly woman with a history of osteoporosis. What changes would you make to your exposure?

2. Your patient is a young woman who is scheduled for a scoliosis series. What should you do in terms of radiation protection for her?

3. When using an AEC device, why is it important to place a lead shield on the tabletop, behind the patient, for a lateral lumbar radiograph?

4. Why is it important to include the kidney shadows on an AP radiograph of the lumbosacral spine?

See page 257 for answers.

SKULL SERIES

Axial (Towne Method)

Requirements

The following must be included on all axial skull radiographs.

SUPERIOR ASPECT. The vertex of the head must be included.

INFERIOR ASPECT. The foramen magnum and base of the skull must be included.

LATERAL ASPECTS. The lateral margins of the skull must be included.

ROTATION. The skull is determined to be not rotated if the distance is equal on both sides of the skull from the foramen magnum to the lateral wall of the skull.

Exposure Critique

DENSITY. Density is acceptable if the bony structures (trabeculae, sutures) in the skull are visually demonstrated.

CONTRAST. Contrast level should be high enough to demonstrate the bony detail within the skull. A mid-kVp range is recommended.

IMAGE DETAIL. The level of detail is acceptable if small structures such as the petrous ridges, posterior clinoid process, and dorsum sella are clearly demonstrated.

DISTORTION. Anatomic structures are deliberately distorted to demonstrate the petrous areas. The distortion is a result of angulation of the central ray.

MAGNIFICATION. Magnification will increase with patient size because of the increase in OID.

SHARPNESS. Motion is present if structures such as the bony trabeculae appear blurred.

ARTIFACTS. The radiograph should be free of artifacts.

Film Identification

Some type of patient identifier, a date and time stamp, and appropriate markers (usually *R* and *L*) should be present on the radiograph.

Critical Film Analysis Form

EXAMINATION ☐

Positioning Critique

Specify the structures that must be included on the radiograph:

Superior Aspect	
Inferior Aspect	
Lateral Aspects	
How would rotation be demonstrated?	

Film Identification	Yes	No
Patient Name/Identifier Present?	☐	☐
Date/Time of Examination Present?	☐	☐
Appropriate Markers Present?	☐	☐

	Yes	No
Evidence of collimation?	☐	☐
Evidence of shielding?	☐	☐

Yes ☐ No ☐

Exposure Factors

		Yes	No
Density	Acceptable?	☐	☐
	Demonstrated by:		
Contrast	Acceptable?	☐	☐
	Demonstrated by:		
Recorded Detail	Acceptable?	☐	☐
	Demonstrated by:		
Distortion	Acceptable?	☐	☐
	Demonstrated by:		
Magnification	Acceptable?	☐	☐
	Demonstrated by:		
Motion Sharpness	Acceptable?	☐	☐
	Demonstrated by:		
Film Artifacts	Acceptable?	☐	☐
	Demonstrated by:		

Posteroanterior

Requirements

The following must be included on all PA skull radiographs.

SUPERIOR ASPECT. The vertex of the skull must be included.

INFERIOR ASPECT. The entire cranial base must be included.

LATERAL ASPECTS. The lateral margins of the skull must be included.

ROTATION. Side-to-side rotation is not present if the distance from the lateral margins of the skull to the outer edge of each orbit is equal. Superior-to-inferior rotation is not present if the petrosa are seen filling the orbital areas.

Exposure Critique

DENSITY. Density is acceptable if the bony structures (trabeculae, sutures) in the skull are visually demonstrated.

CONTRAST. Contrast level should be high enough to demonstrate the bony detail within the skull. A mid-kVp range is recommended.

IMAGE DETAIL. The level of detail is acceptable if small structures such as the petrous ridges, inferior orbital margin, and dorsum sella are clearly demonstrated.

DISTORTION. Distortion should be minimized in the PA projection.

MAGNIFICATION. Magnification will increase with patient size. An AP projection will also increase magnification in structures such as the orbits.

SHARPNESS. Motion is present if structures such as the bony trabeculae appear blurred.

ARTIFACTS. The radiograph should be free of artifacts.

Film Identification

Some type of patient identifier, a date and time stamp, and appropriate markers (usually *R* and *L*) should be present on the radiograph.

Critical Film Analysis Form

EXAMINATION ☐

Positioning Critique

Specify the structures that must be included on the radiograph:

Superior Aspect	
Inferior Aspect	
Lateral Aspects	
How would rotation be demonstrated?	

Film Identification

	Yes	No
Patient Name/Identifier Present?	☐	☐
Date/Time of Examination Present?	☐	☐
Appropriate Markers Present?	☐	☐
Evidence of collimation?	☐	☐
Evidence of shielding?	☐	☐

Yes ☐ No ☐

Exposure Factors

		Yes	No
Density	Acceptable?	☐	☐
	Demonstrated by:		
Contrast	Acceptable?	☐	☐
	Demonstrated by:		
Recorded Detail	Acceptable?	☐	☐
	Demonstrated by:		
Distortion	Acceptable?	☐	☐
	Demonstrated by:		
Magnification	Acceptable?	☐	☐
	Demonstrated by:		
Motion Sharpness	Acceptable?	☐	☐
	Demonstrated by:		
Film Artifacts	Acceptable?	☐	☐
	Demonstrated by:		

Lateral

Requirements

The following must be included on all lateral skull radiographs.

SUPERIOR ASPECT. The vertex of the skull must be included in its entirety.

INFERIOR ASPECT. The base of the skull must be included.

LATERAL ASPECTS. The area from the posterior skull to the entire frontal bone must be included.

ROTATION. Rotation is determined by the demonstration of the sella turcica in profile. The orbital roofs should also be superimposed.

Exposure Critique

DENSITY. Density is acceptable if the bony structures (trabeculae, sutures) in the skull are visually demonstrated.

CONTRAST. Contrast level should be high enough to demonstrate the bony detail within the skull. A mid-kVp range is recommended.

IMAGE DETAIL. The level of detail is acceptable if small structures such as the superimposed air-filled cells of the mastoid processes, the anterior and posterior clinoid processes, and the external acoustic meatus are clearly demonstrated.

DISTORTION. Distortion should be minimal as long as the skull is properly positioned (patient's interpupillary line is perpendicular to the plane of the image receptor and the mid-sagittal plane is parallel to the image receptor) and the alignment of radiographic tube to image receptor is perpendicular.

MAGNIFICATION. The uppermost mandible may be magnified because of the increase is OID.

SHARPNESS. Motion is present if structures such as the bony trabeculae appear blurred.

ARTIFACTS. The radiograph should be free of artifacts.

Film Identification

Some type of patient identifier, a date and time stamp, and appropriate markers (usually *R* and *L*) should be present on the radiograph.

Critical Film Analysis Form

EXAMINATION ☐

Positioning Critique

Specify the structures that must be included on the radiograph:

Superior Aspect	
Inferior Aspect	
Lateral Aspects	
How would rotation be demonstrated?	

Film Identification	Yes	No
Patient Name/Identifier Present?	☐	☐
Date/Time of Examination Present?	☐	☐
Appropriate Markers Present?	☐	☐

	Yes	No
Evidence of collimation?	☐	☐
Evidence of shielding?	☐	☐

Yes ☐ No ☐

Exposure Factors

		Yes	No
Density	Acceptable?	☐	☐
	Demonstrated by:		
Contrast	Acceptable?	☐	☐
	Demonstrated by:		
Recorded Detail	Acceptable?	☐	☐
	Demonstrated by:		
Distortion	Acceptable?	☐	☐
	Demonstrated by:		
Magnification	Acceptable?	☐	☐
	Demonstrated by:		
Motion Sharpness	Acceptable?	☐	☐
	Demonstrated by:		
Film Artifacts	Acceptable?	☐	☐
	Demonstrated by:		

Clinical Challenge

1. Name a pathology that is best demonstrated on a lateral skull radiograph.

2. How would you demonstrate air-fluid levels in the maxillary sinuses?

3. What type of body habitus often requires the placement of a sponge under the patient's chest area when positioning a lateral skull?

4. A patient with a history of vertigo would benefit from which skull positions?

See page 258 for answers.

HAND

Posteroanterior

Requirements

The following must be included on all PA hand radiographs.

SUPERIOR ASPECT. The entire wrist must be included.

INFERIOR ASPECT. The distal ends of all digits must be included.

LATERAL ASPECTS. All fingers and metacarpal areas must be included.

ROTATION. Rotation can be determined if the distal tufts of each finger are *not* equidistant from the sides of the fingernail. The thumb should appear in an oblique position.

Exposure Critique

DENSITY. Density is acceptable if the bony trabeculae and cortex of the bones of the hand are visually demonstrated.

CONTRAST. The range of kVp should be such that the contrast is relatively short. This scale of contrast will provide maximum visibility of anatomic detail such as trabeculae and cortex, and will also demonstrate subtle changes within a fracture.

IMAGE DETAIL. The level of detail is acceptable if details such as bony trabeculae, joint spaces, and distal tufts of the digits are sufficiently demonstrated. A small focal spot should be used to enhance detail. Evidence of collimation should also be present.

DISTORTION. Distortion of all parts of the hand should be minimal, assuming proper alignment of the tube and image receptor.

MAGNIFICATION. Magnification will be minimal in all cases.

SHARPNESS. Motion may be caused by muscle spasms. A radiolucent sponge or other immobilization device may be required to reduce involuntary patient motion.

ARTIFACTS. The radiograph should be free of artifacts such as rings.

Film Identification

Some type of patient identifier, a date and time stamp, and appropriate markers (usually *R* and *L*) should be present on the radiograph.

Critical Film Analysis Form

EXAMINATION ☐

Positioning Critique

Specify the structures that must be included on the radiograph:

Superior Aspect	
Inferior Aspect	
Lateral Aspects	
How would rotation be demonstrated?	

Film Identification	Yes	No
Patient Name/Identifier Present?	☐	☐
Date/Time of Examination Present?	☐	☐
Appropriate Markers Present?	☐	☐

	Yes	No
Evidence of collimation?	☐	☐
Evidence of shielding?	☐	☐

Yes ☐ No ☐

Exposure Factors

		Yes	No
Density	Acceptable?	☐	☐
	Demonstrated by:		
Contrast	Acceptable?	☐	☐
	Demonstrated by:		
Recorded Detail	Acceptable?	☐	☐
	Demonstrated by:		
Distortion	Acceptable?	☐	☐
	Demonstrated by:		
Magnification	Acceptable?	☐	☐
	Demonstrated by:		
Motion Sharpness	Acceptable?	☐	☐
	Demonstrated by:		
Film Artifacts	Acceptable?	☐	☐
	Demonstrated by:		

Oblique

Requirements

The following must be included on all oblique hand radiographs.

SUPERIOR ASPECT. The entire wrist, including the distal ulna and radius, must be included.

INFERIOR ASPECT. The distal ends of all digits must be included.

LATERAL ASPECTS. All digits and metacarpal areas must be included.

ROTATION. Rotation can be deemed minimal if the interphalangeal and metacarpal joint spaces are open.

Exposure Critique

DENSITY. Density is acceptable if the bony trabeculae and cortex of the bones of the hand are visually demonstrated.

CONTRAST. The range of kVp should be such that the contrast is relatively short. This scale of contrast will provide maximum visibility of anatomic detail such as trabeculae and cortex, and will also demonstrate subtle changes within a fracture.

IMAGE DETAIL. The level of detail is acceptable if details such as bony trabeculae, joint spaces, and distal tufts of the digits are sufficiently demonstrated. A small focal spot should be used to enhance detail. Evidence of collimation should also be present.

DISTORTION. Distortion of all parts of the hand should be minimal, assuming proper alignment of the tube and image receptor.

MAGNIFICATION. Magnification will be increased in the uppermost portion of the hand.

SHARPNESS. Motion may be caused by muscle spasms. A radiolucent sponge or other immobilization device may be required to reduce involuntary patient motion.

ARTIFACTS. The radiograph should be free of artifacts such as rings.

Film Identification

Some type of patient identifier, a date and time stamp, and appropriate markers (usually *R* and *L*) should be present on the radiograph.

Critical Film Analysis Form

EXAMINATION ☐

Positioning Critique

Specify the structures that must be included on the radiograph:

Superior Aspect	
Inferior Aspect	
Lateral Aspects	
How would rotation be demonstrated?	

Film Identification	Yes	No
Patient Name/Identifier Present?	☐	☐
Date/Time of Examination Present?	☐	☐
Appropriate Markers Present?	☐	☐

	Yes	No
Evidence of collimation?	☐	☐
Evidence of shielding?	☐	☐

Yes ☐ No ☐

Exposure Factors

		Yes	No
Density	Acceptable?	☐	☐
	Demonstrated by:		
Contrast	Acceptable?	☐	☐
	Demonstrated by:		
Recorded Detail	Acceptable?	☐	☐
	Demonstrated by:		
Distortion	Acceptable?	☐	☐
	Demonstrated by:		
Magnification	Acceptable?	☐	☐
	Demonstrated by:		
Motion Sharpness	Acceptable?	☐	☐
	Demonstrated by:		
Film Artifacts	Acceptable?	☐	☐
	Demonstrated by:		

Lateral

Requirements

The following must be included on all lateral hand radiographs.

SUPERIOR ASPECT. The entire wrist, including the distal ulna and radius, must be included.

INFERIOR ASPECT. The distal ends of the digits must be included.

LATERAL ASPECTS. All digits and metacarpals must be included.

ROTATION. Rotation is minimal if the metacarpals are superimposed. On the fan lateral position, the individual phalanges should be seen with clear delineation of the joint spaces.

Exposure Critique

DENSITY. Density is acceptable if the bony trabeculae and cortex of the bones of the hand are visually demonstrated.

CONTRAST. The range of kVp should be such that the contrast is relatively short. This scale of contrast will provide maximum visibility of anatomic detail such as trabeculae and cortex, and will also demonstrate subtle changes within a fracture.

IMAGE DETAIL. The level of detail is acceptable if details such as bony trabeculae, joint spaces, and distal tufts of the digits are sufficiently demonstrated. A small focal spot should be used to enhance detail. Evidence of collimation should also be present.

DISTORTION. Distortion of all parts of the hand should be minimal, assuming proper alignment of the tube and image receptor.

MAGNIFICATION. Magnification will be increased in the uppermost portion of the hand.

SHARPNESS. Motion may be caused by muscle spasms. A radiolucent sponge or other immobilization device may be required to reduce involuntary patient motion.

ARTIFACTS. The radiograph should be free of artifacts such as rings.

Film Identification

Some type of patient identifier, a date and time stamp, and appropriate markers (usually *R* and *L*) should be present on the radiograph.

Critical Film Analysis Form

EXAMINATION ☐

Positioning Critique

Specify the structures that must be included on the radiograph:

Superior Aspect	
Inferior Aspect	
Lateral Aspects	
How would rotation be demonstrated?	

Film Identification	Yes	No
Patient Name/Identifier Present?	☐	☐
Date/Time of Examination Present?	☐	☐
Appropriate Markers Present?	☐	☐

	Yes	No
Evidence of collimation?	☐	☐
Evidence of shielding?	☐	☐

Yes ☐ No ☐

Exposure Factors

		Yes	No
Density	Acceptable?	☐	☐
	Demonstrated by:		
Contrast	Acceptable?	☐	☐
	Demonstrated by:		
Recorded Detail	Acceptable?	☐	☐
	Demonstrated by:		
Distortion	Acceptable?	☐	☐
	Demonstrated by:		
Magnification	Acceptable?	☐	☐
	Demonstrated by:		
Motion Sharpness	Acceptable?	☐	☐
	Demonstrated by:		
Film Artifacts	Acceptable?	☐	☐
	Demonstrated by:		

Clinical Challenge

1. What is a boxer's fracture?

2. Your patient is a 45-year-old man. You have radiographed his hands before, and this time you notice that his hands do not fit on the average-size cassette. In fact, his hands have grown in size. What should you do?

See page 258 for answers.

FEMUR

Anteroposterior

Requirements

The following must be included on all AP femur radiographs.

SUPERIOR ASPECT. The head of the femur must be included, along with the entire acetabular rim.

INFERIOR ASPECT. The knee joint must be included.

LATERAL ASPECTS. The entire femur must be included, along with greater trochanter and approximately 2 in. of the lateral portion of the inferior ramus of the pubis.

ROTATION. Rotation of the part can be determined when:

- The greater trochanter is not demonstrated in profile.
- More than a small portion of the lesser trochanter is pointing medially.
- Elongation of the femoral neck is not demonstrated.

A patient's femur must never be internally rotated unless the patient is able to do so. Forcing a patient to rotate the femur internally can lead to severe damage in fracture or other serious trauma.

Note: *The entire femur and all soft tissue components must be included.*

Exposure Critique

DENSITY. Density is acceptable if the overall optical density provides optimal visibility of bony detail such as trabeculae.

CONTRAST. The range of kVp should be such that the radiograph exhibits relatively high contrast. A kVp range of 70 to 80 kVp (lower range to mid-range) should provide the necessary visibility of soft tissue structures such as muscle and tendon, as well as sufficient bony detail to visualize fractures.

IMAGE DETAIL. The level of detail is acceptable if details such as soft tissue edema and muscle atrophy are sufficiently demonstrated. A small focal spot should be used to enhance detail. Evidence of collimation should also be present.

DISTORTION. Foreshortening or elongation of anatomical structures should be minimal.

MAGNIFICATION. Magnification will increase with patient size because of the increase in OID.

SHARPNESS. Motion may be caused by muscle spasms. A sandbag or sponge may be required to reduce involuntary patient motion.

ARTIFACTS. Lead shielding should be evident on the radiograph. It should not obscure areas of interest.

Film Identification

Some type of patient identifier, a date and time stamp, and appropriate markers (usually *R* and *L*) should be present on the radiograph.

Critical Film Analysis Form

EXAMINATION ☐

Positioning Critique

Specify the structures that must be included on the radiograph:

Superior Aspect	
Inferior Aspect	
Lateral Aspects	
How would rotation be demonstrated?	

Film Identification	Yes	No
Patient Name/Identifier Present?	☐	☐
Date/Time of Examination Present?	☐	☐
Appropriate Markers Present?	☐	☐

	Yes	No
Evidence of collimation?	☐	☐
Evidence of shielding?	☐	☐

Yes ☐ No ☐

Exposure Factors

		Yes	No
Density	Acceptable?	☐	☐
	Demonstrated by:		
Contrast	Acceptable?	☐	☐
	Demonstrated by:		
Recorded Detail	Acceptable?	☐	☐
	Demonstrated by:		
Distortion	Acceptable?	☐	☐
	Demonstrated by:		
Magnification	Acceptable?	☐	☐
	Demonstrated by:		
Motion Sharpness	Acceptable?	☐	☐
	Demonstrated by:		
Film Artifacts	Acceptable?	☐	☐
	Demonstrated by:		

Lateral

Requirements

The following must be included on all lateral radiographs of the femur.

SUPERIOR ASPECT. A lateral image of the femoral head in the acetabulum must be included. This requires a cross-table lateral radiograph of the hip.

INFERIOR ASPECT. A lateral image of the superimposed femoral condyles, including the patella, must be included.

LATERAL ASPECTS. The entire femur and soft tissue must be included.

ROTATION. Rotation will not be present if the patella is seen in profile.

Note: *A cross-table lateral femur should be used in cases of trauma, recent surgery of the femur, or fracture.*

Exposure Critique

DENSITY. Density is acceptable if the overall optical density provides optimal visibility of bony detail such as trabeculae.

CONTRAST. The range of kVp should be such that the radiograph exhibits relatively high contrast. A kVp range of 70 to 80 kVp (lower range to mid-range) should provide the necessary visibility of soft tissue structures such as muscle and tendon, as well as sufficient bony detail to visualize fractures. An additional lateral radiograph of the hip may be be necessary. This is required because of the density differences between the femur and hip areas.

IMAGE DETAIL. The level of detail is acceptable if details such as soft tissue edema and muscle atrophy are sufficiently demonstrated. A small focal spot should be used to enhance detail. Evidence of collimation should also be present.

DISTORTION. If the anatomic structures are represented correctly on the radiograph, distortion can be said to be minimal. If a cross-table lateral radiograph is taken, the femoral neck should be parallel to the grid and the central ray should be perpendicular to the femoral neck and grid. Failure to achieve this will result in grid cutoff and increased distortion.

MAGNIFICATION. Magnification will increase with patient size because of increased OID.

SHARPNESS. Motion may be caused by muscle spasms. If patients are positioned so that they are turned onto the affected femur, the use of radiographic sponges or sandbags is recommended.

ARTIFACTS. Lead shielding should be evident on the radiograph. It should not obscure areas of interest.

Film Identification

Some type of patient identifier, a date and time stamp, and appropriate markers (usually *R* and *L*) should be present on the radiograph.

Critical Film Analysis Form

EXAMINATION ☐

Positioning Critique

Specify the structures that must be included on the radiograph:

Superior Aspect	
Inferior Aspect	
Lateral Aspects	
How would rotation be demonstrated?	

Film Identification	Yes	No
Patient Name/Identifier Present?	☐	☐
Date/Time of Examination Present?	☐	☐
Appropriate Markers Present?	☐	☐

	Yes	No
Evidence of collimation?	☐	☐
Evidence of shielding?	☐	☐

Yes ☐ No ☐

Exposure Factors

		Yes	No
Density	Acceptable?	☐	☐
	Demonstrated by:		
Contrast	Acceptable?	☐	☐
	Demonstrated by:		
Recorded Detail	Acceptable?	☐	☐
	Demonstrated by:		
Distortion	Acceptable?	☐	☐
	Demonstrated by:		
Magnification	Acceptable?	☐	☐
	Demonstrated by:		
Motion Sharpness	Acceptable?	☐	☐
	Demonstrated by:		
Film Artifacts	Acceptable?	☐	☐
	Demonstrated by:		

Clinical Challenge

1. Describe the shielding that you could provide for the patient requiring femur radiographs.

2. What is a giant cell tumor and how does it appear radiographically?

3. Your patient requires a portable radiograph of the femur. How do you decide if you should use a grid or not?

See page 258 for answers.

ANSWERS TO THE CLINICAL CHALLENGE QUESTIONS

Chest

1. Both inspiration and expiration PA chest radiographs would be required if there is a question of a foreign body (e.g., peanut in the bronchus) and in cases of pneumothorax.
2. The position of the patient is helpful to radiologists during interpretation of the radiographs. A patient in the supine position would not be able to take as deep a breath as one in the erect position. The SID must also be marked to allow the radiologist to compensate for magnification of the heart and great vessels. Patients who have portable chest radiographs may have more than one radiograph per day. Therefore, all portable radiographs must have a time marker on them as well. This allows the physician to determine the order in which the radiographs were taken.
3. You should write a note to the radiologist stating that the radiograph was correctly labeled (assuming that you have indeed marked it correctly).
4. Yes. Portable chest radiographs on infants require a nongrid technique. Consequently, low kVp is used. The blanket will show up as an artifact. It may be a better idea to warm up the cassette by placing it under your laboratory coat for a while. Also, keep in mind that young patients wear flame-retardant pajamas, which may also cause artifacts.
5. No. The central ray should be directed parallel with the floor. This will demonstrate the presence of interlobar effusions. The position of the patient, SID used, and time of the radiograph should be noted, as well as the fact that the central ray was parallel to the floor.

Abdomen (Anteroposterior)

1. An AP projection, with the patient in the left lateral decubitus position, would be used. This position demonstrates the presence of fluid and air levels and is used so that any free air present will rise to the uppermost portion of the abdomen, which is the right side. The liver is also on this side, and it provides an excellent backdrop for free air. Fluid, on the other hand, will fall to the patient's left side. It is extremely important that the patient be placed in this position for several minutes before making an exposure. This allows the fluid and air to fall or rise to the appropriate sides.
2. If the patient has ascites sufficient enough to distend his abdomen, an increase in kVp would be needed to penetrate the ascites. The increase in kVp would be determined by measuring the area in question.
3. You should plan on producing two radiographs. One radiograph would be placed transverse and positioned to include the upper portion of the abdomen. The other radiograph, which would also be placed transverse, would be positioned to include the pelvic area. You should first align the patient so that the entire body is in the same place (shoulders in the same plane as pelvis). Palpate for the xiphoid process. If you cannot locate the xiphoid, center the midpoint of the cassette midway between the level of the breasts. For the second exposure, position the second cassette so that there would be an overlap of approximately 2 in. with the first exposure. Another means of determining the position of the two cassettes is to place the bottom of one cassette approximately 2 in. below the iliac crest and the top of the second cassette 2 in. above the iliac crest.
4. If the radiologist is unable to determine what these microcalcifications are, then slight oblique radiographs of the area may be requested. These would require a small focal spot and close collimation. Depending on the equipment

used, mAs may need to be increased up to four times what was used to produce the 14 × 17 inch abdomen radiograph.

GI Series

1. Place the patient in either the RAO or the right lateral position. If possible, have the patient walk around, or have the patient talk to you about his or her favorite foods.
2. The duodenal bulb and pyloric canal.
3. Air and barium should be located as follows:
   - AP: Air would be across the body of the stomach; barium would be in the fundus.
   - PA: Air would be in the fundus; barium would be in the body of the stomach.
   - Right lateral: Air would in the fundus; barium would be in the body of the stomach.
   - RAO: Air would be in the fundus; barium would be in the body of the stomach, in the pylorus, and in the duodenum.
   - LPO: Air would be across the body of the stomach; barium would be in the fundus. If the patient is left in this position, air will rise to the pylorus as well.

Barium Enema

1. The AP axial projection can be substituted.
2. Lateral rectum and axial Chasshand-Lapine projections may be used.
3. The splenic flexure is not included.
4. High kVp exposure is used for a regular, or single, barium enema study because it facilitates barium penetration, giving the radiologist more information. If the kVp exposure is low, the barium will appear as a large white area, providing little or no visualization of the anatomic detail within.

Cervical Spine

1. The AEC device has not been placed directly over the cervical spine. Instead, the chamber is placed over the soft tissue of the neck, resulting in a radiograph that is underexposed.
2. The spinous process of the lower cervical or upper thoracic spine is involved.
3. The AP cervical spine projection will demonstrate the cervical ribs.
4. An AP axial projection should be taken for the vertebral arch. This requires the patient to be supine and to hyperextend his or her neck. The central ray is directed approximately 20 degrees caudal. This position demonstrates the lateral masses of the vertebrae.

Lumbosacral Spine

1. Although you may be tempted to increase your kVp because of the patient's size, a history of osteoporosis tells you that the patient's bones are demineralized. To demonstrate this condition, you must keep your kVp as low as possible and increase your mAs appropriately.
2. You should do the following:
   - Make certain that the patient is not pregnant.
   - Shield the patient's gonadal region.
   - Shield the patient's breasts.
   - Place the patient in the PA position to reduce the exposure to both the breast area and the gonads.
   - Use close collimation.
   - Use a rare earth screen system and high kVp technique.

3. A lead shield absorbs scatter radiation coming from the patient. When using an AEC device, the exposure can be terminated because of this scatter radiation, resulting in an underexposed radiograph. Close collimation should always be used.
4. Including the kidney area may assist the physician in interpretation of the radiograph. A patient who has back pain may also have a kidney stone. Keep in mind that not all kidney stones are radiopaque. A radiolucent stone may cause hydronephrosis, which may be seen as an enlarged kidney shadow.

Skull Series

1. An enlarged sella turcica caused by pituitary enlargement may be seen. Paget's disease is also commonly seen on lateral skull radiographs as well as AP pelvis radiographs.
2. An erect parietoacanthial projection, Water's method, would demonstrate this condition. If the patient is not able to sit or stand, a horizontal central ray projection, taken with the patient supine and using close collimation, may be helpful.
3. Hyposthenic or asthenic body habitus requires the placement of a sponge.
4. The axial skull position, which demonstrates the petrous areas that house the inner ear, should be used. The second choice would be a PA skull position, which would demonstrate the petrous areas seen within the orbits. A third choice would be an axiolateral oblique projection (posterior profile), Stenvers method. This demonstrates the petrous ridges in profile.

Hand

1. Fracture of the neck of the fifth metacarpal, with palmar deviation, is a boxer's fracture. A clenched fist striking a hard object commonly causes this.
2. Use a larger cassette, of course. However, it is more important to inform the physician. An adult's hands do not normally grow larger, and this could be caused by acromegaly. Acromegaly, which is caused by hyperpituitarism, starts after the bones have stopped growing. Other clinical symptoms include enlargement of the face and soft tissues.

Femur

1. Initial radiographs should demonstrate as much of the adjacent areas as possible. This should include the area of the acetabulum and as much of the pelvis as possible. Gonadal shielding should be used when information will not be lost because of the placement of the shield. A lead shield can be placed over the ovary areas of female patients. Male patients should wear a lead glove on one hand and gently move the scrotal sac to the opposite side.
2. This is a benign condition commonly seen in young adults. It is commonly seen in the distal femur. Radiographically, it appears as large bubbles, separated by bone.
3. The common rule is, if the part measures 10 cm or more, use a grid.

References

1. Bushong, SC: Radiologic Science for Technologists, ed 6., Mosby-Year Book, Inc. St. Louis, 1997, p 230.
2. Ibid, p 230
3. Ibid, p 260
4. Ibid, p 265
5. Ibid, p 265
6. Ibid, p 269
7. Ibid, p 269

8. Ibid, p 240
9. Ibid, pp 245–246
10. Ibid, p 420
11. Ibid, p 420
12. Ibid, p 421
13. Ibid, pp 422–423
14. Drafke, MW: Trauma and Mobile Radiography, F. A. Davis, Philadelphia, 1990, pp 111–112.

Bibliography

Bushong, SC: Radiologic Science for Technologists, ed 6. Mosby-Year Book, Inc. St. Louis, 1997.
Drafke, MW: Trauma and Mobile Radiography, F. A. Davis, Philadelphia, 1990.

Critical Thinking Outcome Assessment

PURPOSE

The form that follows is designed to demonstrate the graduating student's ability in applying critical thinking skills within the clinical setting. It is intended as a synopsis of all the student's work.

It is recommended that the graduating student include this form, with all appropriate signatures and seals, in his or her resumé, which will be sent to prospective employers.

DIRECTIONS

The program director and clinical instructor will evaluate and mark the appropriate areas of the Critical Thinking Outcome Assessment Form. The program director and clinical instructor should ensure that the student has adequate documentation to support the data on the form.

Critical Thinking Outcome Assessment Form

Graduating Student's Name ______________________ Date __________

This form demonstrates the graduating student's successful application of critical thinking skills in the following areas:

Part A. GENERAL

	Acceptable	Very Good	Exceptional
Positioning factors	_____	_____	_____
Patient care factors	_____	_____	_____
Ethical conduct	_____	_____	_____
Radiographic exposure factors	_____	_____	_____
Radiation protection practices	_____	_____	_____
Pathologies	_____	_____	_____
Organizational skills	_____	_____	_____
Leadership skills	_____	_____	_____
Communication skills	_____	_____	_____
Patient assessment	_____	_____	_____

Part B. CRITICAL ANALYSIS OF RADIOGRAPHS

	Acceptable	Very Good	Exceptional
Positioning	_____	_____	_____
Exposure factors	_____	_____	_____
Radiation protection	_____	_____	_____
Film identification	_____	_____	_____

Part C. MODIFICATION OF STANDARD PROCEDURE FOR PATIENT FACTORS

	Acceptable	Very Good	Exceptional
Pathology	_____	_____	_____
Patient history	_____	_____	_____
Patient ability	_____	_____	_____
Patient age	_____	_____	_____
Portable radiography	_____	_____	_____
Patient body habitus	_____	_____	_____
Radiographic equipment	_____	_____	_____
Professional growth and development	_____	_____	_____

School name ______________________________

Instructor's signature ______________________________

Instructor's title ______________________________

Program director's signature ______________________________

Graduate signature ______________________________

School seal or stamp

____

Index